T0215835

Fast Facts on **ADOLESCENT HEALTH FOR NURSING AND HEALTH PROFESSIONALS**: A Care Guide *(Herrman)*

Fast Facts for the **ANTEPARTUM AND POSTPARTUM NURSE**: A Nursing Orientation and Care Guide *(Davidson)*

Fast Facts Workbook for **CARDIAC DYSRHYTHMIAS AND 12-LEAD EKGs** *(Desmarais)*

Fast Facts for the **CARDIAC SURGERY NURSE**: Caring for Cardiac Surgery Patients, Third Edition *(Hodge)*

Fast Facts for **CAREER SUCCESS IN NURSING**: Making the Most of Mentoring *(Vance)*

Fast Facts for the **CATH LAB NURSE** *(McCulloch)*

Fast Facts for the **CLASSROOM NURSING INSTRUCTOR**: Classroom Teaching *(Yoder-Wise, Kowalski)*

Fast Facts for the **CLINICAL NURSE LEADER** *(Wilcox, Deerhake)*

Fast Facts for the **CLINICAL NURSE MANAGER**: Managing a Changing Workplace, Second Edition *(Fry)*

Fast Facts for the **CLINICAL NURSING INSTRUCTOR**: Clinical Teaching, Third Edition *(Kan, Stabler-Haas)*

Fast Facts on **COMBATING NURSE BULLYING, INCIVILITY, AND WORKPLACE VIOLENCE**: What Nurses Need to Know *(Ciocco)*

Fast Facts for the **CRITICAL CARE NURSE**, Second Edition *(Hewett)*

Fast Facts About **CURRICULUM DEVELOPMENT IN NURSING**: How to Develop and Evaluate Educational Programs, Second Edition *(McCoy, Anema)*

Fast Facts for **DEMENTIA CARE**: What Nurses Need to Know, Second Edition *(Miller)*

Fast Facts for **DEVELOPING A NURSING ACADEMIC PORTFOLIO**: What You Really Need to Know *(Wittmann-Price)*

Fast Facts for **DNP ROLE DEVELOPMENT**: A Career Navigation Guide *(Menonna-Quinn, Tortorella Genova)*

Fast Facts About **EKGs FOR NURSES**: The Rules of Identifying EKGs *(Landrum)*

Fast Facts for the **ER NURSE**: Emergency Department Orientation, Third Edition *(Buettner)*

Fast Facts for **EVIDENCE-BASED PRACTICE IN NURSING**: Third Edition *(Godshall)*

Fast Facts for the **FAITH COMMUNITY NURSE**: Implementing FCN/Parish Nursing *(Hickman)*

Fast Facts About **FORENSIC NURSING**: What You Need to Know *(Scannell)*

Fast Facts for the **GERONTOLOGY NURSE**: A Nursing Care Guide *(Eliopoulos)*

Fast Facts About **GI AND LIVER DISEASES FOR NURSES**: What APRNs Need to Know *(Chaney)*

Fast Facts About the **GYNECOLOGICAL EXAM**: A Professional Guide for NPs, PAs, and Midwives, Second Edition *(Secor, Fantasia)*

Fast Facts in **HEALTH INFORMATICS FOR NURSES** *(Hardy)*

Fast Facts for **HEALTH PROMOTION IN NURSING**: Promoting Wellness *(Miller)*

Fast Facts for Nurses About **HOME INFUSION THERAPY**: The Expert's Best Practice Guide *(Gorski)*

Fast Facts for the **HOSPICE NURSE**: A Concise Guide to End-of-Life Care, Second Edition *(Wright)*

Fast Facts for the **L&D NURSE**: Labor & Delivery Orientation, Second Edition *(Groll)*

Fast Facts for the **LONG-TERM CARE NURSE**: What Nursing Home and Assisted Living Nurses Need to Know *(Eliopoulos)*

Fast Facts to **LOVING YOUR RESEARCH PROJECT**: A Stress-Free Guide for Novice Researchers in Nursing and Healthcare *(Marshall)*

Fast Facts for **MAKING THE MOST OF YOUR CAREER IN NURSING** *(Redulla)*

Fast Facts for **MANAGING PATIENTS WITH A PSYCHIATRIC DISORDER**: What RNs, NPs, and New Psych Nurses Need to Know *(Marshall)*

Fast Facts About **MEDICAL CANNABIS AND OPIOIDS**: Minimizing Opioid Use Through Cannabis *(Smith, Smith)*

Fast Facts for the **MEDICAL OFFICE NURSE**: What You Really Need to Know *(Richmeier)*

Fast Facts for the **MEDICAL–SURGICAL NURSE**: Clinical Orientation *(Ciocco)*

Fast Facts for the **NEONATAL NURSE**: A Nursing Orientation and Care Guide *(Davidson)*

Fast Facts About **NEUROCRITICAL CARE**: A Quick Reference for the Advanced Practice Provider *(McLaughlin)*

Fast Facts for the **NEW NURSE PRACTITIONER**: What You Really Need to Know, Second Edition *(Aktan)*

Fast Facts for **NURSE PRACTITIONERS:** Practice Essentials for Clinical Subspecialties *(Aktan)*

Fast Facts for the **NURSE PRECEPTOR:** Keys to Providing a Successful Preceptorship *(Ciocco)*

Fast Facts for the **NURSE PSYCHOTHERAPIST:** The Process of Becoming *(Jones, Tusaie)*

Fast Facts About **NURSING AND THE LAW:** Law for Nurses *(Grant, Ballard)*

Fast Facts About the **NURSING PROFESSION:** Historical Perspectives *(Hunt)*

Fast Facts for the **OPERATING ROOM NURSE:** An Orientation and Care Guide, Second Edition *(Criscitelli)*

Fast Facts for the **PEDIATRIC NURSE:** An Orientation Guide *(Rupert, Young)*

Fast Facts Handbook for **PEDIATRIC PRIMARY CARE:** A Guide for Nurse Practitioners and Physician Assistants *(Ruggiero, Ruggiero)*

Fast Facts About **PRESSURE ULCER CARE FOR NURSES:** How to Prevent, Detect, and Resolve Them *(Dziedzic)*

Fast Facts About **PTSD:** A Guide for Nurses and Other Health Care Professionals *(Adams)*

Fast Facts for the **RADIOLOGY NURSE:** An Orientation and Nursing Care Guide, Second Edition *(Grossman)*

Fast Facts About **RELIGION FOR NURSES:** Implications for Patient Care *(Taylor)*

Fast Facts for the **SCHOOL NURSE:** What You Need to Know, Third Edition *(Loschiavo)*

Fast Facts About **SEXUALLY TRANSMITTED INFECTIONS:** A Nurse's Guide to Expert Patient Care *(Scannell)*

Fast Facts for **STROKE CARE NURSING:** An Expert Care Guide, Second Edition *(Morrison)*

Fast Facts for the **STUDENT NURSE:** Nursing Student Success *(Stabler-Haas)*

Fast Facts About **SUBSTANCE USE DISORDERS:** What Every Nurse, APRN, and PA Needs to Know *(Marshall, Spencer)*

Fast Facts for the **TRAVEL NURSE:** Travel Nursing *(Landrum)*

Fast Facts for the **TRIAGE NURSE:** An Orientation and Care Guide, Second Edition *(Visser, Montejano)*

Fast Facts for the **WOUND CARE NURSE:** Practical Wound Management *(Kifer)*

Fast Facts for **WRITING THE DNP PROJECT:** Effective Structure, Content, and Presentation *(Christenbery)*

Forthcoming FAST FACTS Books

Fast Facts for the **ADULT-GERONTOLOGY ACUTE CARE NURSE PRACTITIONER** *(Carpenter)*

Fast Facts About **COMPETENCY-BASED EDUCATION IN NURSING:** How to Teach Competency Mastery *(Wittmann-Price, Gittings)*

Fast Facts for **CREATING A SUCCESSFUL TELEHEALTH SERVICE:** A How-to Guide for Nurse Practitioners *(Heidesch)*

Fast Facts About **DIVERSITY, EQUITY, AND INCLUSION** *(Davis)*

Fast Facts for the **ER NURSE:** Guide to a Successful Emergency Department Orientation, Fourth Edition *(Buettner)*

Fast Facts for the **L&D NURSE:** Labor & Delivery Orientation, Third Edition *(Groll)*

Fast Facts About **LGBTQ CARE FOR NURSES** *(Traister)*

Fast Facts for the **NEONATAL NURSE:** Care Essentials for Normal and High-Risk Neonates, Second Edition *(Davidson)*

Fast Facts for the **NURSE PRECEPTOR:** Keys to Providing a Successful Preceptorship, Second Edition *(Ciocco)*

Fast Facts for **PATIENT SAFETY IN NURSING** *(Hunt)*

Visit www.springerpub.com to order.

FAST FACTS for
THE NEONATAL NURSE

Michele R. Davidson, PhD, RN, CNM, PMHNP-BC, PMH-C, CFN, SANE, is currently a psychiatric mental health nurse practitioner and a certified nurse midwife at Leva Psychiatry In Virginia Beach, Virginia, where she specializes in women's mental health and perinatal mood disorders. Dr. Davidson has published over 50 papers, contributed more than 35 chapters to other authors' textbooks, and coauthored an additional 33 textbooks, including the international bestseller, *Old's Maternal–Newborn Nursing and Women's Health Care Across the Lifespan* (10th ed.), which has been translated into 12 languages and used throughout the world. In 2012, Dr. Davidson published *A Nurse's Guide to Women's Mental Health Care,* which earned an AJN Award in psychiatric mental health nursing.

FAST FACTS for
THE NEONATAL NURSE

A Care Guide for Normal and High-Risk Neonates

Second Edition

Michele R. Davidson, PhD, RN, CNM, PMHNP-BC,
PMH-C, CFN, SANE

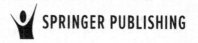

Springer Publishing Company, LLC
11 West 42nd Street, New York, NY 10036
www.springerpub.com
connect.springerpub.com/

Acquisitions Editor: Rachel X. Landes
Compositor: Amnet Systems

ISBN: 978-0-8261-8484-9
ebook ISBN: 978-0-8261-8491-7

DOI: 10.1891/9780826184917

20 21 22 23 / 5 4 3 2 1

Library of Congress Cataloging-in-Publication Data

Names: Davidson, Michele R., author.
Title: Fast facts for the neonatal nurse : care essentials for normal and
  high-risk neonates / Michele R. Davidson.
Other titles: Fast facts (Springer Publishing Company)
Description: Second edition. | New York, NY : Springer Publishing Company,
  LLC, 2020. | Series: Fast facts | Includes bibliographical references
  and index. |
Identifiers: LCCN 2020027528 (print) | LCCN 2020027529 (ebook) | ISBN
  9780826184849 (paperback) | ISBN 9780826184917 (ebook)
Subjects: MESH: Neonatal Nursing—methods | Perinatal Care—methods |
  Infant, Newborn, Diseases—nursing
Classification: LCC RJ253 (print) | LCC RJ253 (ebook) | NLM WY 157.3 |
  DDC 618.92/01—dc23
LC record available at https://lccn.loc.gov/2020027528
LC ebook record available at https://lccn.loc.gov/2020027529

For my children,
Hayden, Chloe, Caroline, and Grant Davidson.
For the four people in this world I hold in my heart and who
have given me the pleasure of watching them learn,
grow, and succeed in this world.
It is hard to believe as you approach this stage of your life,
I am closer to holding grandchildren than I was to
snuggling those four little babies I once sang softly to sleep.
May your lives continue to bring out the best in you, foster your strength,
nurture your enthusiasm, and bring you life's greatest joys!
I could not be prouder that I have four amazing human beings
that I wholeheartedly adore who call me "Mom."

Contents

Part IX PROMOTING HEALTHY FAMILIES IN THE COMMUNITY

Preface

This book provides a basic reference for nurses caring for newborns and high-risk newborns as well as care considerations for families. Nurses continue to function as valued members of a collaborative healthcare team, play a primary role in the assessment and care of the newborn, and provide education for new parents regarding the newborn's needs. Families experience dramatic transformations as roles develop and change during the newborn period, and rely on the knowledge, support, and encouragement of the nurse to learn to care for their newborn and meet the newborn's most basic needs. In-depth knowledge of the physiological changes of the newborn enables the nurse to detect possible complications that warrant additional assessment. Early identification of risk factors and complications can help ensure that proper newborn evaluation and care are provided when alterations are present.

Advancements in obstetrical care practices have led to advances and options for very premature newborns. Infants who would not have survived if born decades earlier now have far greater chances of survival, though some will have lifelong consequences as a result of birth occurring at early gestational ages. Although most births occur at term and without serious complications, 11.5% of newborns are born prematurely (before 37 completed weeks). Prematurity remains the greatest risk factor for newborn morbidity and mortality. Prematurity is also the leading cause of disabilities in children.

In acute care facilities, it is the nurse who performs the initial newborn assessment and obtains measurements and other assessment data. A thorough knowledge of normal newborn characteristics enables the competent nurse to quickly identify deviations from normal characteristics or potential complications. If an abnormality is identified, it is the nurse's role to notify the clinician and initiate interventions to ensure that stabilization of the newborn is promptly achieved. Most abnormalities, birth defects, or complications are identified during the newborn examination.

The nurse plays an invaluable role in providing education to the family on the proper care of the newborn, including assisting with feedings. Breastfeeding is the preferred method of feeding for all infants, regardless of gestational age. The American Academy of Pediatrics recommends exclusive breastfeeding for the first 6 months of life. Successful and long-term breastfeeding has been noted to be highest in women who receive initial breastfeeding opportunities as soon as possible after birth with assistance from educated nurses who can provide hands-on support. The nurse assists the mother in learning basic provisions for infant feeding and supports the mother's choice of feeding method. Some women will opt not to breastfeed and continue to need guidance and education to ensure proper nutrition for the newborn.

Although the vast majority of infants are born without long-term complications, some newborns experience short-term complications. Although these conditions are short term in nature, they do require immediate intervention and treatment. Cold stress, hypoglycemia, jaundice, respiratory distress, fluid and electrolyte conditions, and infections are usually not associated with long-term complications if they are identified early and promptly treated. Other complications have ongoing implications that may require more intensive interventions and longer treatment durations, such as prematurity or low birth weight. A small number of infants will be born with conditions that have lifelong implications and may require intensive care or management strategies, such as genetic defects or birth defects.

Although most nurses face ethical dilemmas in practice, the newborn nursery nurse, especially the neonatal intensive care unit nurse, faces these on a regular basis. Infants may be exposed to the mothers' substance abuse and alcohol use in pregnancy, which can have lifelong consequences. Other infants are born on the edge of viability and will require intensely complex decisions to determine the most ethical and compassionate plan of care. Some of these newborns will require emergency procedures, whereas some of these newborns will need transport to obtain life-saving measures. Other newborns will have conditions that are incompatible with life, leaving families facing harrowing issues of death and dying. Any family faced with unexpected birth outcomes, whether birth trauma, injury, or previously unidentified disorders, needs extensive support, education, and compassion.

Newborns face multiple vulnerabilities and need specialized care from their caregivers in order to establish normal growth and development and to prevent illness and injury. Nurses must possess excellent communication skills and have knowledge of various procedures and care needs, such as immunizations, proper sleeping positions, fall precautions, and travel recommendations. Nurses give explanations in order to provide comprehensive holistic teaching to families about the initial care for the newborn in the home environment. Ongoing educational needs include the need for newborn examinations, well visits in the infant period, and infant immunizations.

The nurse caring for the newborn also provides a great deal of support and has extensive interaction with the mother and the family. Support for the postpartum family includes identifying potential risk factors, providing referrals for community support groups, and referral to appropriate multidisciplinary providers, such as pediatric providers or lactation support specialists. The nurse also has extensive interactions with the new mother and should perform postpartum depression and mood and anxiety disorders (PMAD) screening. Approximately 20% of new mothers will develop postpartum depression, which can negatively impact the family, including the newborn. Prompt identification and treatment are associated with better outcomes. Care of the mother with a PMAD includes referral to support groups, evaluation by a skilled practitioner for possible pharmacological interventions, and a multidisciplinary approach that includes skilled professionals. Women leaving the hospital without their infant may be at risk for postpartum depression and require additional support related to their individualized circumstances.

There is no greater joy, responsibility, honor, or blessing than to be afforded the opportunity to work with growing families at this amazing time in their expanding lives. Each newborn and family is entirely unique, different, and, in some way, utterly amazing. There are those who will pass through a nurse's life uneventfully, and although it is almost sad to say, will likely be forgotten, blending in with the many memories that merge together in the days that will eventually create the weeks, months, and years that knit together a nursing career.

Many nurses caring for newborns likely take for granted that sweet baby smell, the smooth skin against your cheek, or the time spent in rockers quieting fussy newborns back to sleep. The daily tasks of life for a nurse can become mundane and repetitive, but it is my greatest hope that you will embrace each newborn and each new family who comes under your care. For nurses who have their own children, it is likely that, as with your own newborn experience, these days will eventually slip away as you move to a different patient care area or transition into retirement, and you will be left reminiscing about your days spent in a nursery rocking chair or feeding a new-born whose mother is sound asleep from a long exhaustive labor. It is quite likely that when that time comes, you will miss those days as a neonatal nurse. It is my hope that actively practicing nurses will enjoy and appreciate each and every newborn encounter and that the families you help will permanently imprint themselves on your heart and soul, providing you with vivid memories. I hope each day continues to instill in you a passion that inspires you to wake up with anticipation, providing you with the reason to continue to care for families during this crucial time period in their lives!

Michele R. Davidson

Acknowledgments

When I was a new graduate nurse, I worked in the postpartum setting and the newborn nursery, and now realize it is the best nursing job there is! Later, I became a certified nurse midwife and was blessed to deliver over a thousand babies and care for thousands more families during that time. Although I loved delivering babies, it is those quiet nights sitting in rocking chairs in a downtown Washington, D.C., hospital that I remember most vividly and with the fondest of memories. Throughout that time, I am not sure I was aware of the sacred gift that I had been provided, or that I truly valued the many tremendous experiences encountered, or how much I would miss those snuggly newborns when my career path moved forward. For all the families who shared their precious newborns with me and allowed me to care for their most valued life's treasures, my genuine thanks to you!

Although I rejoiced with many families during perhaps the happiest moments in their lives, I was also privileged to care for newborns facing the greatest of challenges. I have had several newborns die in my arms because their parents couldn't bear to watch them take their last breath. It was many of those families who in their darkest hours shared the most intimate and raw feelings of human heartache that have shaped my philosophy of nursing and of life and ignited my desire to provide compassionate care to all families as they navigate both the joys and heartaches that often come with having a baby. It is with immense thanks and gratitude that I would like to acknowledge all of those families for providing me with the opportunity to share their joys and tears.

Special thanks to my husband, Nathan Davidson, CFNP, who also provided support and expertise in content. His unending support and encouragement are always appreciated and valued. My mom, Geri Lewis, is always my best cheerleader and provides support and encouragement, and is a true mentor of this crazy role I call "motherhood."

My own personal experience with newborns lies with having the absolute joy of bringing home four beautiful babies, Hayden, Chloe, Caroline, and Grant, who have taught me more in their young lives than any professional education or professor could ever provide. My youngest child, Grant, was born at 30 gestational weeks and suffered spastic quadriplegia, giving me direct personal experience with unexpected birth outcomes, which over the years has enabled me to possess a greater understanding of the absolute critical need for empathy, resilience, and hope—critical attributes that families facing these unique challenges truly need. My son is a child who illustrates incredible personal strength, presents with remarkable courage, and never gives up; he chooses to conquer life's struggles with grace, persistence, and determination. He has taught me a great deal about the experiences of unexpected outcomes, birth defects, and losses faced by some parents. He is truly a blessing who has been an inspiration not only to me, but to everyone who has encountered him in his or her life's journey. Our journey and his life are a testament to how one learns from life's greatest challenges and finds the silver lining in what seems like life's gravest events!

I

Newborn Physiology and Initial Newborn Exams, Assessments, and Procedures

1

Physiological Adaptations to Birth

The newborn undergoes drastic physiological changes at the time of birth. The neonatal transition period begins at the time of birth, with the respiratory and circulatory system transitions occuring immediately. While the vast majority of newborns in the United States transition smoothly, approximately 10% will require some intervention, and 1% will require intensive resuscitation. Other systems may take longer to become fully functional after birth. The nurse provides ongoing observation and performs frequent assessments during this period to ensure underlying pathological alterations are not present that could interfere with the newborn's successful adaptation to extrauterine life.

During the neonatal transition period, the nurse will be able to:

1. Identify normal and abnormal assessment findings in the newborn.
2. Describe the changes required by each body system for successful adaptation to extrauterine life.
3. Discuss the respiratory and cardiovascular changes that occur during the transition to extrauterine life and during stabilization.
4. Identify the advantages of delayed cord blood clamping.
5. Describe how various factors affect the newborn's blood values.
6. Understand the steps involved in excretion of bilirubin in the newborn and discuss the reasons a newborn may develop jaundice.
7. Describe the functional ability of the newborn's liver and gastro-intestinal tract.

8. Discuss reasons a newborn's kidneys have difficulty maintaining fluid and electrolyte balance.
9. List the immunologic responses of the newborn.
10. Describe the normal sensory abilities and behavioral states of the newborn.

RESPIRATORY SYSTEM

Physiology of the Respiratory System

- The development of the respiratory system in utero begins with the differentiation of structures into pulmonary, vascular, and lymphatic structures. The embryonic stage begins at 4 to 5 weeks with the formation of the larynx, trachea, and bud branches, which will later form the left and right lung. The pseudoglandular phase occurs up until 17 weeks; during this phase, buds develop from the trachea and form independent bronchioles surrounded by capillaries that will later enable oxygen extention. Fetal breathing movements, in utero practice respiratory movements, begin by 17 to 20 weeks.
- The canalicular phase occurs between 18 and 25 weeks, enabling respiratory capillary formation where the air–blood barrier develops, which enables oxygen inhalation and carbon dioxide exhalation within the capillaries Beginning at 20 weeks, alveolar ducts develop.
- By the third trimester, the final physiological changes occur that are essential for independent breathing in extrauterine life. By 24 to 28 weeks, alveoli differentiate into type I cells, which aid in gas exchange, and type II cells, which produce and store surfactant. At 28 to 32 weeks, surfactant production significantly increases, aiding the lungs' ability to expand, which is vital for extrauterine respiration.

Physiological Adaptations Following Birth

- Initiation of neonatal breathing at birth

  - Although the lungs are still filled with fluid at the time of birth, lung fluid production decreases 24 to 26 hours prior to birth.
  - Lung expansion occurs at the time of birth.
  - An increase in pulmonary circulation occurs as a result of increased oxygen levels within the neonatal lungs. Blood flow resistance also decreases.

- Mechanical stimuli

  - Fetal gasp occurs within 10 seconds of expulsion and is initiated by a central nervous system trigger in response to the sudden change in pressure and temperature.
  - Fetal chest compression and chest recoils occur during expulsion.
  - With neonatal exhalation and crying against a partially closed glottis, positive intrathoracic pressure occurs.
  - Fluid is absorbed into the lymphatic system and capillaries as lung expansion occurs, moving oxygen into the bloodstream while carbon dioxide is exhaled.

- Chemical stimuli

  - Transitory asphyxia occurs due to:
    - Increases in PCO_2
    - Decreases in pH and PO_2
    - Stimulation of the aortic and carotid chemoreceptors triggers the respiratory system in the medulla.
    - Prostaglandin levels drop when the cord is cut.

- Other stimuli

  - Changes in temperature stimulate skin sensors and rhythmic respirations.
  - Environmental components include tactile, auditory, visual, and pain stimuli.

Indicators of Initial Normal Functioning

- Respiratory rate of 30 to 60 breaths/minute
- Diaphragmatic breathing
- Periodic breathing with apnea periods of 5 to 10 seconds may occur
- Initially shallow
- Irregular in depth and rhythm
- Pulse oximetry levels >95%

Fast Facts

Newborns born via cesarean birth may have an increased amount of fluid in their lungs; thus, observation for neonatal transition is necessary and additional bulb suctioning is required.

Indicators of Abnormal Functioning

- Respiratory rate less than 30 or greater than 60 breaths/minute
- Irregular depth (persistently shallow) and irregular rhythm
- Nasal flaring
- Chest retractions
- Generalized cyanosis
- Apnea periods >20 seconds associated with cyanosis
- Apnea associated with bradycardia
- A single pulse oximetry measurement <90%
- Pulse oximetry <95% on the right hand and either foot on three different measures, each 1 hour apart

Fast Facts

The newborn is an obligatory nose breather and any obstruction can lead to respiratory distress; it is essential that the nurse monitor for any signs of distress.

CARDIOVASCULAR SYSTEM

Physiology of the Cardiovascular System

- Cardiovascular development begins to occur within 3 weeks of the mother's last menstrual period (LMP); circulation begins and the structure of the heart begins to form.
- By 4 weeks, the tubular heart beats (by 22 to 23 days) and blood flow begins (28 days, post-LMP) as circulation between the fetus and placenta occurs; detection of the fetal heart rate, however, typically does not occur until 6 to 7 weeks.
- Atrial division occurs at 5 weeks, and the chambers are clearly defined by 6 weeks.
- By 8 weeks, the heart is fully formed and functioning.

Physiological Adaptations Following Birth

- The initial breath at birth decreases pulmonary vascular resistance, increasing blood flow to the lungs.
- Blood returning from the pulmonary veins increases pressure in the right atrium.

- When the umbilical cord is clamped, umbilical venous blood flow stops completely, dropping pressure in the right atrium and increasing systemic vascular resistance.
- Complete transition from fetal circulation to neonatal cardiopulmonary adaptation involves multiple processes (Table 1.1).

Table 1.1

Physiological Cardiac Changes From Fetal to Newborn Circulatory System

Physiological Shift in Cardiac Functioning	Physiological Process That Occurs With Change
Increased aortic pressure	Umbilical cord clamping reduces the intravascular space and halts perfusion to the umbilical cord.
Decreased venous pressure	Aortic blood flow increases, which accommodates the systemic circulatory needs.
	Blood flow to the inferior vena cava decreases.
	Decreased right atrial pressure occurs.
	Small reduction in venous circulation occurs.
Increased systemic pressure	Increase in systemic pressure with circulation no longer needed for the placenta
Decreased pulmonary artery pressure	Lung expansion increases pulmonary circulation as the pulmonary blood vessels dilate, which decreases pulmonary artery resistance.
	Systemic vascular pressure increases to increase systemic perfusion.
Closure of foramen ovale	Closure occurs with a shift in the arterial pressure, which stops the shunting of blood between atria.
	Right atrial pressure drops in response to decreasing vascular resistance and increased pulmonary blood flow.
	Functional closure of the foramen ovale occurs after birth at 1–2 hours of age; however, complete closure does not occur until approximately 30 months.
	During crying, hypothermia, cold stress, hypoxia, or acidosis, the foramen ovale could reopen, causing a right-to-left shunt to occur.

(continued)

Table 1.1

Physiological Cardiac Changes From Fetal to Newborn Circulatory System (*continued*)	
Physiological Shift in Cardiac Functioning	**Physiological Process That Occurs With Change**
Closure of the ductus arteriosus	Pulmonary vascular pressure increases pulmonary blood flow by reversing the blood flow through the ductus arteriosus.
	Increased levels of oxygen cause the ductus arteriosus to constrict.
	Functional closure occurs 10–15 hours after birth, with complete closure occurring by 4 weeks.
Closure of the ductus venosus	Mechanical pressures occur when the umbilical cord is clamped, blood is redistributed, and cardiac output increases, resulting in blood flow to the liver.
	Functional closure occurs within 2 months.

Indicators of Initial Normal Functioning

- Color at birth should be pink or reddish-pink with acrocyanosis being common in the first 5 minutes following birth.
- Initial cardiac rate is 110 to 180 beats per minute (bpm) but can be as high as 180 due to initial crying effort.
- Resting heart rate between 110 and 160 bpm
- During certain activity periods, bpm can vary:

  - Deep sleep state can be as low as 80 to 100 bpm
  - Active awake state can be up to 180 bpm

- Regular rhythm and rate
- Point of maximum impulse located on left side of chest (indicating correct anatomical position)
- Peripheral pulses should be palpable and bilaterally equal, although pedal pulses may be difficult to palpate.
- The capillary refill time is 2 to 3 seconds.
- Blood pressure (BP) tends to be higher immediately after birth and then decreases by around 3 hours of age. It rises and stabilizes within 4 to 7 days to the approximate initial level reached immediately after birth. The average mean BP is 42 to 60 mmHg in the resting full-term newborn over 3 kg.

- Systolic heart murmurs may be present as the circulation transfers from a fetal to neonatal state and are usually due to the incomplete closure of the ductus arteriosus or foramen ovale.

Indicators of Initial Abnormal Functioning

- Point of maximum impulse on right side of chest (indicating abnormal anatomical position)
- Cardiac rates less than 110 or above 180 bpm
- Cardiac arrhythmias
- Abnormal heart sounds (split second heart sound, gallops, ejection clicks, and diastolic murmurs)
- Heart rate less than 90 bpm that does not increase with stimulation (heart block)
- Irregular rate and rhythm
- Reduction in upper extremity pulses (poor cardiac output or peripheral vasoconstriction)
- Absence of pedal pulses (poor cardiac output or peripheral vasoconstriction)
- Prolonged capillary refill time of greater than 4 seconds
- Blood pressure with a gradient >10% in systolic blood pressure measurements between upper and lower extremities
- Abnormal color (paleness could indicate anemia while ruddy red color could indicate polycythemia)
- Cyanosis
  - Cyanosis is momentarily relieved by crying (choanal atresia)

Delayed Umbilical Cord Clamping

- Delayed cord clamping is defined as delaying the clamping of the cord for at least 1 minute or until the cord has stopped pulsating and is now the recommended standard of care for infants not needing resuscitation.
- Benefits term and preterm infants
- No maternal risks
- Higher serum hemoglobin concentrations at 24 to 48 hours of life
- Higher birth weight
- Fewer neonatal blood transfusions
- Increased iron stores at 3 to 6 months of age
- Reduction of intraventricular brain hemorrhage
- Reduction in necrotizing enterocolitis
- Increased incidence of phototherapy for jaundice

Physiology of the Hematological System

- Hematopoiesis refers to the differentiation of the blood cell components within the hematological system and is divided into three stages: mesoblastic, hepatic, and myeloid.
- During fetal development, rudimentary blood moves through primitive vessels connecting to the yolk sac and chorionic membranes at 7 gestational weeks.
- The arterial system develops mainly from the aortic arches.
- The venous system emerges from three bilateral veins and is completed by the eighth gestational week.

Physiological Adaptations Following Birth

- Increase in catecholamines results in increased cardiac output required for maintaining increased metabolic oxygen needs related to thermogenesis, breathing, and feeding demands.
- Fetal right-sided dominance switches to left-sided dominance by 3 to 6 months of age.
- Fetal hemoglobin (HgF) is replaced with adult hemoglobin (HgA) by 6 months of age. The hemoglobin levels decline during the first 2 months of life, leading to a phenomenon known as physiological anemia of the newborn. The lowest hemoglobin level occurs around 3 months of age and is called the physiologic nadir.

Normal Newborn Laboratory Values

- Red blood cell (RBC) production and survival are lower in the newborn than in adults. The average neonatal RBC has a life span of 60 to 80 days (two-thirds of the life span of adult RBCs).
- Normal blood volume ranges from 80 to 90 mL/kg
- White blood cell (WBC) counts rangefrom 10,000 to 30,000/mm^3, with polymorphonuclear leukocyte (PMN) predominance.
- Iron stores will be used to produce new RBCs, which means most infants will require supplemental iron to maintain adequate iron stores.

  - By the 6 months, bone marrow has become the chief site of blood formation.

- Leukocytosis is a normal finding due to the stress of birth and the subsequent increased production of neutrophils during the first few days of life. Neutrophils then decrease by around 2 weeks of age.
- Blood volume varies based on the amount of placental volume received during delivery. It can be altered by delayed cord

clamping, gestational age, prenatal or perinatal hemorrhage, and the site of lab draw on the newborn.

- Electrolyte values change based on the age of the newborn (Table 1.2).

Fast Facts

Keep in mind the reference ranges from your own laboratory.

- Glucose 40 to 60 mg/dL for first 24 hours, then 50 to 90 mg/dL
- Low blood sugar of 40 to 45 mg/dL requires treatment.

Fast Facts

Hemoglobin levels in the newborn fall primarily due to a decrease in red blood cell mass rather than from an increase in plasma volume, causing a dilution.

- Vitamin K-dependent clotting factors (II, XII, IX, X) become active.

Fast Facts

The initial administration of a vitamin K injection protects against prolonged bleeding until the newborn's liver begins to function adequately and establishes normal clotting factors.

HEPATIC SYSTEM

Physiology of the Hepatic System

- Human liver development begins during the third week of gestation; however, it is not fully mature until around 15 years of age. It reaches its largest relative size, about 10% of fetal weight, around the ninth week gestation and constitutes about 5% of body weight in the healthy full-term neonate.

Table 1.2

Blood Electrolyte Values for Term Infants

Value	Cord	1–12 hours	12–24 hours	24–48 hours	48–72 hours	>3 days
Sodium (mEq/L)	147 (126–166)	143 (124–156)	145 (132–159)	148 (134–160)	149 (139–162)	—
Potassium (mEq/L)	7.8 (5.6–12)	6.4 (5.3–7.3)	6.3 (5.3–8.9)	6.0 (5.2–7.3)	5.9 (5.0–7.7)	—
Chloride (mEq/L)	103 (98–110)	101 (80–111)	103 (87–114)	102 (92–114)	103 (93–112)	—
Calcium (mmol/L)	2.33 (2.1–2.8)	2.1 (1.8–2.3)	1.95 (1.7–2.4)	2.0 (1.5–2.5)	1.98 (1.5–2.4)	—
Calcium (mmol/24 hours)	—	1.05–1.37	1.05–1.37	1.05–1.37	1.10–1.44	1.20–1.48
Phosphate (mmol/L)	1.8 (1.2–2.6)	1.97 (1.1–2.8)	1.84 (0.9–2.6)	1.91 (1.0–2.8)	1.87 (0.9–2.5)	—
Magnesium (mmol/L)	—	—	0.72–1.00	—	0.81–1.05	0.78–1.02
Urea (mmol/L)	10.4 (7.5–14.3)	9.6 (2.9–12.1)	11.8 (3.2–22.5)	11.4 (4.6–27.5)	11.1 (5.4–24.3)	—
Creatinine (mmol/L)	—	—	—	0.04–0.11	—	0.01–0.09
C-reactive protein (mg/L)	<7	<7	<7	<7	<7	<7
Lactate (mmol/L)	1.5–4.5	0.9–2.7	0.8–1.2	—	—	0.5–1.4
Albumin (g/L)	28–43	28–43	28–43	28–43	28–43	30–43
Alkaline phosphatase (IU/L)	28–300	28–300	28–300	28–300	28–300	28–300
Thyroid-stimulating hormone	—	—	3.0–120	3.0–30	—	0.3–10

Cortisol (nmol/L)	200–700	200–700	200–700	200–700	—	—
17-hydroxyprogesterone (nmol/L)	—	—	—	—	0.7–12.4	0.7–12.4
Hemoglobin (g/L)	168	—	—	184	178	170
Hematocrit (%)	53	—	—	58	55	54
Mean corpuscular volume	107	—	—	108	99	98
Reticulocytes (%)	3–7	—	—	3–7	1–3	0–1
White cell count 3 10^9/L	18.1 (9–30)	22.8 (13–38)	18.9 (9.4–34)	—	—	12.2 (5–21)
Neutrophils 3 10^9/L	11.1 (6–26)	15.5 (6–28)	11.5 (5–21)	—	—	5.5 (1.5–10)
Lymphocytes 3 10^9/L	5.5 (2–11)	5.5 (2–11)	5.8 (2–11.5)	—	—	5.0 (2–17)
Monocytes 3 10^9/L	1.1	1.2	1.1	—	—	1.1
Eosinophils 3 10^9/L	0.4	0.5	0.5	—	—	0.5
Platelets (10^3/mm^3)	150–350	150–350	150–350	150–350	150–350	150–350
Prothrombin time (seconds)	—	11–14	11–14	11–14	11–14	11–14
Activated partial thromboplastin time (seconds)	—	23–35	23–35	23–35	23–35	23–35

Physiological Adaptations Following Birth

The newborn's liver plays a vital role in the following processes:

- Iron storage for new RBC production

  - Prenatally, if the mother's iron intake has been adequate, there is enough iron stored to last 5 months. At around 6 months of age, food containing iron and/or iron supplements must be added to the infant's diet.

- Coagulation

  - The absence of normal flora needed to synthesize vitamin K results in low levels of vitamin K and creates a transient blood coagulation alteration between the second and fifth days after birth.

- Carbohydrate metabolism

  - The newborn's cord blood glucose level is 15 mg/dL lower than the maternal blood glucose level. The newborn's carbohydrate reserve is relatively low. During the first 2 hours of life, the serum blood glucose level declines and then begins to rise, reaching a steady state by about 3 hours. If the fetus experiences hypoxia or stress, the glycogen stores are used and may be depleted. Glucose is the main source of energy in the first 4 to 6 hours of life.

- Conjugation of bilirubin

  - Conjugation is the conversion of bilirubin from the yellow fat-soluble, unconjugated/indirect form into a water-soluble, excretable/direct form.

    - Unconjugated bilirubin (fat soluble) is a potential toxin that is not an excretable form of bilirubin and must be conjugated (made water soluble) to be excreted from the body.

  - Unconjugated bilirubin is a breakdown product derived from the heme portion of hemoglobin that is released from destroyed RBCs.

  - Physiological jaundice occurs after the first 24 hours of life.

    - Physiological hyperbilirubinemia is a buildup of bilirubin due to the normal hemolysis of red blood cells needed for fetal circulation before birth and it is discarded afterward. The imbalance of an immature liver and an overabundance of bilirubin to process allows the yellow pigment from hemolyzed red cells to accumulate in the blood and gives the skin and sclera the yellow tone we call *jaundice*.

❑ About 50% of all infants exhibit signs of jaundice in the 2 to 3 days after birth due to decreased glucuronyl transferase.

■ Pathological jaundice occurs before 24 hours of life.

❑ Pathological hyperbilirubinemia is related to a condition other than normal newborn bilirubin being processed slowly by an immature liver. Such conditions include incompatibility between the newborn's and the mother's blood types, incompatibility of additional blood factors, or liver problems. These above mentioned conditions are pathologies that may require more aggressive and lengthier treatments.

Fast Facts

In utero, the fetus lives in a state of relative hypoxia, with a PaO_2 of approximately 35 mmHg, compared to 80 mmHg for a healthy child or adult. To maximize the oxygen-carrying capacity of the blood, the fetus produces more RBCs, with a hematocrit level up to 60 being normal.

At birth, the newborn's PaO_2 increases. The excess RBCs are no longer needed for oxygen-carrying capacity and begin to break down. This normal, physiologic change occurs at birth. The breakdown of these RBCs releases bilirubin into the bloodstream.

If something causes an excessive number of RBCs to break down (such as ABO or Rh incompatibility, birth trauma, or infection) or impairs the newborn's ability to pass bilirubin out of the gastrointestinal tract (nothing orally [NPO], delayed stooling, or meconium ileus), the bilirubin level rises. Delayed cord clamping can increase the number of RBCs and lead to an increase in bilirubin levels. Bilirubin levels at birth are about 3 mg/dL and should not exceed 12 mg.

Fast Facts

Nursing care should include keeping the newborn well hydrated and promoting early and frequent elimination. Early feedings tend to keep bilirubin levels down by stimulating intestinal activity, thus removing the contents and not allowing reabsorption.

GASTROINTESTINAL SYSTEM

Physiology of the Gastrointestinal System

- In utero, fetal swallowing, gastric emptying, and intestinal peristalsis occur. By the end of gestation, peristalsis is much more active in preparation for extrauterine life. Fetal peristalsis is also stimulated by anoxia, and low oxygen states in utero (postterm, placental insufficiency, fetal stress, umbilical cord compromise) can cause a premature meconium stool in utero.
- By 36 to 38 weeks of fetal life, the gastrointestinal (GI) system is sufficiently mature to support extrauterine life.

Fast Facts

Digestion of protein and carbohydrates is adequate. However, fat digestion and absorption are poor due to the absence of adequate pancreatic enzymes.

Physiological Adaptations Following Birth

- The newborn's stomach holds about 50 to 60 cc and can pass meconium 24 to 48 hours after birth.
- Permeability—The newborn's intestines lack the protective mucosal barrier that helps seal off the intestines, decreasing the risk of both bacteria and potential allergens permeating through the intestine into the bloodstream.
- Digestive enzymes—The newborn pancreas does not produce the enzymes, such as amylase, needed to digest complex carbohydrates or starches until around the age of 3 months. Newborns also produce less lipase during the first year of life.
- The lower esophageal sphincter is still immature and therefore opens more easily than it will later in life. This allows a small amount of food to reflux up. Infants who fail to gain weight due to a large amount of reflux should be further evaluated for gastroesophageal reflux disease.

Indicators of Initial Normal Functioning

- There is a normal physiologic weight loss in the newborn of around 6% to 10% (loss of body water) due to:
  - Diuresis

- Expulsion of meconium
- Withholding of water and calories

- The newborn should gain between .5 to 1 ounce per day, double the birth weight by 5 to 6 months of age, and triple the birth weight by 1 year of age.
- The normal newborn's pattern of elimination

  - Stools—Meconium is stool that contains epithelial cells, bile, and amniotic fluid. In 90% of normal newborns, meconium stools occur within 24 hours of life. This is a black, tarry stool that will transition to brownish green. Transitional stools are part meconium and part fecal stool from the digestion of milk. Formula-fed infants will pass two to three bright-yellow stools per day that may appear "seedy" and may have a strong odor, depending on the type of formula. Breastfed infants will pass several small, light-yellow stools per day with little or no odor. Formula-fed infants' bowel movements (BMs) will be the consistency of toothpaste, whereas breastfed infants' BMs will remain quite loose as there is little that is not digested. A newborn who does not pass meconium within 24 to 48 hours of birth should be examined for the possibility of imperforate anus, meconium ileus, bowel obstruction, or cystic fibrosis. Infants with acholic stools (gray or clay-colored stools) need to undergo a workup for liver abnormalities (Hansen, Eichenwald, Stakr, & Martin, 2016).

URINARY SYSTEM

Physiology of the Kidneys and Urinary System

- Urine production occurs in utero as early as the fourth month, and there are functioning nephrons by 34 to 36 weeks gestation. The glomerular filtration rate of the newborn's kidney is low. The ability to concentrate and dilute urine is attained by 3 months of age; however, before that, monitoring of fluid therapy to prevent overhydrating or dehydration is necessary.

Physiological Adaptations Following Birth

- Many newborns void immediately after birth, with about 90% voiding by 24 hours of life. A newborn who has not voided by 48 hours of life should be evaluated for adequacy of fluid intake or urinary/bladder abnormality or dysfunction.
- Normal urine is straw colored and odorless.

- In the first 2 days of life, the newborn will void two to six times a day, with a urine output of 15 mg/kg/day. Subsequently, the newborn will void between 6 and 25 times every 24 hours, with a urine output of 25 mg/kg/day.
- Following the initial void, the newborn's urine is frequently cloudy due to mucus and a high specific gravity. Pink-stained urine, called "brick dust spots," will occasionally be seen. These are caused by urates and are harmless.
- Blood may also be observed on the diapers of female newborns. Pseudomenstruation is related to the maternal withdrawal of hormones.
- Persistent dark urine could indicate a build-up of bilirubin, possibility indicating liver disease.

IMMUNOLOGICAL SYSTEM

Physiology of the Immune System

- The newborn's immune system is not initiated until after birth. Due to the newborn's limited inflammatory response, there is a failure to recognize and therefore respond to bacteria. This is why the signs and symptoms of infection in the newborn are often subtle and nonspecific.
- Of the three major types of immunoglobulins (IgG, IgA, IgM), only IgG can cross the placenta. Newborns have what is termed *passive acquired immunity* against viruses to which the mother had antibodies (diphtheria, poliomyelitis, measles, mumps, varicella, tetanus, rubella, smallpox) as a result of maternal IgG that crossed the placenta. These passive maternal immunoglobulins are primarily transferred during the third trimester of pregnancy. Therefore, preterm infants may be more susceptible to infection (Gomella, Eyal, & Bany-Mohammed, 2020).
- Passive immunity is also acquired during breastfeeding. During breastfeeding, maternal antibodies, white blood cells, enzymes, and immune factors, are transferred to the newborn which helps strengthen the immune system.
- Although newborns can produce or mount a response to antigens and begin development of antibodies, their immunity is not as effective as an older child's. Because of this, it is customary to wait to begin the majority of routine immunizations until 2 months of age, when the infant can develop *active acquired immunity* more efficiently.

Fast Facts

Active acquired immunity—the mother forms antibodies in response to illness or immunization. *Passive acquired immunity*—transfer of immunoglobulins to the fetus in utero (IgG production begins at 20 weeks gestation) or to the infant via breast milk.

Physiological Adaptations Following Birth

Fast Facts

There is little immunity to herpes simplex virus (HSV), so caretakers with an active HSV infection need to wear a mask and gloves.

NEUROLOGICAL SYSTEM

Physiology of the Neurological System

- By 3 gestational weeks, the fetal brain has differentiated into the forebrain, midbrain, and hindbrain, and begins functioning by 4 gestational weeks. By the end of 8 weeks, the internal organs and their connection with the brain are functioning
- Rapid growth of the fetal brain occurs during the last half of fetal life, peaking near the time of birth, with a pronounced acceleration in the eighth month.

Physiological Adaptations Following Birth

Babies move through several transition periods in the first 6 hours after birth as their systems change and stabilize.

First alert period: (15–30 minutes after birth) Baby is alert, respirations are irregular, responds vigorously to stimulation

Resting period: (30–120 minutes after birth) Color and vital signs are stabilizing, baby sleeps and is difficult to arouse

Second alert period: (4–8 hours after birth) Awakening, becoming responsive to stimuli again, may have a lot of mucus to clear

■ Behavioral States

1. Quiet sleep	Deep sleep, no eye movement, respirations are quiet and slower
2. Active sleep	Rapid eye movements, may move extremities or stretch
3. Drowsy	Transitional period, yawns, eyes glazed
4. Quiet alert	Infant able to focus on objects or people, tuned in to environment
5. Active alert	Restless, starting to fuss, faster respirations, more aware of discomfort

The newborn's response to stimuli is simple.

■ Senses

Touch	This is the most significant sense in the newborn for the first few weeks of life.
Vision	Newborns can see objects 8 to 12 inches from their eyes. Newborns are most drawn to faces, particularly the eyes. They are able to follow objects to center of visual field. They prefer yellow and red objects and will regard moving objects and changing light intensity.
Hearing	The newborn will turn toward the sound of a voice and tends to be more alert to a high-pitched voice.
Taste	They are able to discriminate between sweet/nonsweet.
Smell	The newborn's ability to smell increases over the first few days of life. The newborn is able to identify the mother's breast milk.

Indicators of Initial Normal Functioning

Newborn or infant reflexes are reflexes that are normal in infants but abnormal in other age groups.

■ Primitive reflexes are present at the time of birth and are brainstem-mediated, automatic movements.

■ Primitive reflexes begin to develop around 25–26 gestational weeks and continue to develop until the time of birth.

■ In very preterm infants, the development of these reflexes could be impaired or not yet developed.

■ Persistently weak, overly exaggerated, or unsymmetrical responses could be a sign of neurological impairment.

Normal newborn reflexes include:

Reflex	Description
Moro	Infant's head is gently lifted and then released suddenly, falling backward for a moment. The normal response is for the baby to have a startled look, and arms should move sideways with the palms up and thumbs flexed. The baby may cry for a minute.
Suck	Sucks when the area around the mouth is touched.
Startle	Pulls arms and legs in after hearing a loud noise.
Step	Makes stepping motions when the sole of the foot touches a hard surface.
Tonic neck (fencing position)	When you move the head of a child who is relaxed and lying on his back to the side, the arm on the side where the head is facing reaches straight away from the body with the hand partly open. The arm on the side that is away from the face is flexed and the fist is clenched tightly. Turning the baby's face in the other direction reverses the position.
Galant (truncal incurvation)	Occurs when you stroke or tap along the side of the spine while the infant lays on the stomach. The infant will twitch his or her hips toward the touch in a back-and-forth motion.
Grasp	Occurs if you place a finger on the infant's open palm. The hand will close around the finger. Trying to remove the finger causes the grip to tighten.
Rooting	When you stroke the infant's cheek, the infant will turn toward the side that was stroked and begin to make sucking motions.
Parachute	Occurs in slightly older infants; when you hold the child upright and then rotate his or her body quickly to face forward (as if falling), the baby will extend his or her arms forward.
Blinking	Blinks eyes when the eyes are touched or when a sudden bright light appears.
Cough	Coughs when the airway is stimulated.
Gag	Gags when the throat or back of the mouth is stimulated.
Sneeze	Sneezes when the nose is stimulated.
Yawn	Yawns when the body needs more oxygen.

References

Gomella, T., Eyal, F., & Bany-Mohammed, F. (2020). *Gomella's neonatology: Management, procedures, on-call problems, and drugs*. Philadelphia, PA: McGraw-Hill Education.

Hansen, A. R., Eichenwald, E. C., Stakr, A. R., & Martin, C. R. (2016). *Cloherty & Stark's manual of neonatal care* (8th ed.). St. Louis, MO: Lippincott, Williams, & Wilkins.

2

Initial Newborn Procedures and Assessments

The initial newborn examination is performed immediately after birth to detect any gross abnormalities and identify issues associated with the transition to extrauterine life. Immediately after birth, the nurse performs a test to determine an Apgar score, which indicates how the newborn is adapting and ensures that essential vital functions are operating. The nurse ensures proper temperature regulation and provides a neutral thermal environment for the newborn. An assessment is also performed to determine the infant's gestational age. Gestational age assessment is used to determine whether the newborn has any risk factors related to prematurity. Assessments during the first 24 hours after birth provide essential information and ensure the newborn is appropriately adapting to the new external environment. The nurse conducts multiple procedures during this time period to ensure a smooth transition during the newborn period.

During this part of the orientation, the nurse will be able to:

1. Identify components of the initial newborn examination that is performed during the first hour after birth.
2. List the variables assessed in Apgar scoring.
3. Discuss interventions for maintaining a neutral thermal environment immediately following birth.
4. Describe the importance of a gestational age assessment.

5. Define the appropriate intervals for newborn assessments during the first 24 hours after birth.
6. Identify critical procedures that should be performed in the first 24 hours after birth.

INITIAL NEWBORN EXAMINATION

The initial newborn examination is performed at the time of birth, typically as soon as possible after the newborn has been stabilized but no more than 2 hours after birth. The exam is performed in the birthing room at the maternal bedside unless maternal or newborn complications are present.

➡ High Risk Care

A generalized overall assessment for congenital defects or chromosomal disorders should be performed on all newborns at the time of birth. While any infant can have a previously unknown risk for a genetic or congenital birth defect, some infants will be identified as high risk prior to the onset of labor. Risk factors for congenital birth defects include (Hansen, Eichenwald, Stakr, & Martin, 2016):

- Mothers with advanced maternal age
- Family history of congenital or genetic defects
- Previous sibling born with a known defect or genetic abnormality
- Maternal history of stillbirth of unknown etiology
- Abnormal prenatal screening test results
- Presence of abnormal ultrasound findings
- Infants born to diabetic mothers

Routine Assessment for Anomalies or Abnormalities

- Observe for the presence of three vessels in the cut end of the umbilical cord. When a single umbilical artery is present, the risk of birth defects is 15% to 20%.
- Inspect the palms for a single simian crease, which is associated with chromosomal defects, including Down syndrome.
- Observe for facial asymmetry and dysphoric features, which can be indicative of congenital malformations.
- Inspect eyes for upward or downward slanting and/or an epicanthic fold, eye position, which can be an indicator of a genetic abnormality.
- Inspect position of ears and size of ears, as smaller-than-expected ear size and low-set ears can be associated with chromosomal defects.
- Inspect mouth, tongue, nose, and nasal bridge formation, for normal appearance. A flat nose, smaller-than-expected

mouth, and protruding tongue can be signs of Down syndrome.

- Inspect for webbing of the neck, fingers, and toes as well as thespace between the first and second toe, as this can be associated with genetic abnormalities.
- Observe crying that appears asymmetrical, as this can indicate hypoplasia of the depressor angularis oris muscle.
- Close inspection of proper formation, location, and patency of all body orifices should be made to determine if potential congenital defects are present.
- Conduct Apgar scoring at 1 minute and 5 minutes.
- Respiratory assessment

  - Complete a visual inspection for symmetry with circular chest with equal anteroposterior and lateral diameter
  - Assess for symptoms of respiratory distress (tachypnea, bradypnea, irregular respiratory rate, retractions, nasal flaring, cyanosis).
  - Auscultation of lungs
  - Respiratory rate and rhythm (irregular respirations are normal) should be monitored for 60 full seconds.

- Cardiac evaluation

  - Heart rate should be monitored for 60 full seconds.
  - Heart rhythm
  - Presence of abnormalities (murmurs, gallops, clicks, extra heart sounds)
  - Cyanosis

- Vital sign assessment

  - Heart rate of 110 to 160 bpm
  - Respirations of 30 to 60 breaths/minute
  - Temperature: 97.5 to 99°F (36.0 to 37.2°C)
  - Blood pressure: 70–50/45–30 mmHg

- Umbilical cord assessment (three vessels with Wharton's jelly covering the cord; bleeding, redness, and signs of infection should not be present; cord clamp placed correctly with no skin pinched in clamp)

NEWBORN RESUSCITATION AT TIME OF BIRTH

Newborn resuscitation is warranted when a normal transition with adequate respirations, heart rate, and normal circulation has not been established. Approximately 10% of newborns will need some resuscitation, with only 1% needing intensive efforts. Initial methods of stabilization include:

- Dry newborn, providing stimulation for initial breath.
- Term infants with vigorous crying and good muscle tone should be placed on mother's chest for stabilization.
- Preterm infants, infants without crying or breathing efforts, or those with poor tone should be placed on radiant warmer.
- Provide warmth under radiant warmer.
- Clear airway only if necessary and position head upright in a sniffing position.
- Assess respirations (a crying newborn has adequate respiration; apnea, gasping, or labored breathing may warrant ventilation).
- Evaluate heart rate simultaneously using the umbilical pulse; rates with a bpm of 100 or lower warrant intervention.

➡ High Risk Care

Any newborn may need resuscitation at the time of birth, but some newborns can be identified as high risk for resuscitation prior to birth because of known placental, maternal or fetal or intrapartum risk factors. Anticipating resuscitation can help staff, providers, and parents prepare for the procedures that may be needed to assist the newborn(s) to transition to extrauterine life (Gomella, Eyal, & Bany-Mohammed, 2020).

Placental Factors

- Placenta previa
- Abruptio placentae
- Abnormal cord insertions (velamentous cord insertion, vasa previa)
- Intrapartum bleeding
- Reduced placenta perfusion
- Prolonged pregnancy
- Postterm pregnancy

Maternal Factors

- Gestational hypertension, preeclampsia, eclampsia
- Hemolysis, elevated liver enzymes, low platelet count (HEELP) syndrome
- Autoimmune Disease
- History of assisted reproductive Ttchnology
- Intrahepatic cholestasis
- Thrombophilia

- Pregestational diabetes or gestational diabetes
- Severe renal insufficiency
- Advanced maternal age
- Substance abuse (alcohol, tobacco, illicit drugs)
- Previous pregnancy complications
- Excessive stress, mental health disorders
- Obesity
- Malnutrition
- Polyhydramnios
- Oligohydramnios
- Nongynecoid pelvis type or pelvis with narrowing bone structure
- Maternal thyroid disorder
- Maternal fever
- Maternal hypoglycemia
- Maternal hypothermia
- Maternal hypotension or hypoxia
- Preexisting infectious disease (HIV, hepatitis B or C, HSV, CMV)
- Cephalopelvic disproportion
- Lack of prenatal care
- Poverty
- Maternal age (>35 or <20 years)
- Anaphylactoid syndrome of pregnancy
- Uterine rupture
- Rh incompatibility

Fetal Factors

- Chromosomal or genetic anomalies
- Intrauterine growth restriction
- Multiple gestation
- Macrosomia
- Preterm gestation
- Cardiac defects
- Passage of meconium

Intrapartum Factors

- Nonreassuring fetal status
- Prolonged labor
- Induced or augmented labor
- Prolonged second stage
- Cesarean birth
- Vacuum or forceps (instrument-assisted) birth
- Shoulder dystocia

- Unfavorable antepartum testing (nonreactive non-stress test [NST], abnormal biophysical profiles [BPP] or abnormal modified biophysical profile [MBP], abnormal Doppler studies in high-risk pregnancies, positive contraction stress test [CST])
- Abnormal category 2 intrapartum fetal heart rate tracings (sinusoidal pattern, bradycardia, tachycardia, arrhythmias, tachysystole, lack of variability)
- Malpresentation (acynclitism, breech [in singleton birth or in second twin], face, brow, compound, occiput posterior)
- Umbilical cord prolapse
- Labor dystocia
- Precipitous labor and birth
- Metabolic acidosis
- Administration of sympatholytics, parasympatholytics, or general anesthesia
- External cephalic version with labor induction immediately following
- Uteroplacental insufficiency
- Birth asphyxia
- Prolonged rupture of membranes
- Group beta streptococcal infection

Resuscitation Procedure

When neonatal distress occurs, resuscitation measures may be warranted. Initial resuscitation involves:

- Evaluate airway.
- Clear the airway via suctioning as needed.
- If poor respiratory functioning is present, positive pressure ventilation (PPV) with an Ambu bag is begun at 40 to 60 breaths/minute.
- If heart rate is less than 60 bpm after 30 seconds of PPV, chest compressions are warranted.
- If the heart rate remains less than 60 bpm despite adequate ventilation (usually with endotracheal intubation) and 100% oxygen and chest compressions, administration of epinephrine or volume expansion, or both, may be indicated.
- Buffers, a narcotic antagonist, or vasopressors may be useful after resuscitation, but these are not recommended in the delivery room and are rarely needed.
- Typical resuscitation efforts are maintained for 10 minutes before termination is considered.

NEUTRAL THERMAL ENVIRONMENT

A neutral thermal environment is one in which the newborn maintains his or her current temperature without using body reserves. Heat production in the neonate is via metabolism and nonshivering thermogenesis. Brown fat, which develops by 28 gestational weeks, insulates the newborn and allows for thermogenesis to take place.

Infants at Risk for Heat Loss and Hypothermia (See also Table 2.1)

- Premature infants
- Infants with sepsis
- Infants with central nervous system injuries or anomalies
- Small-for-gestational-age infants
- Prolonged resuscitation efforts

Interventions to Prevent Heat Loss

Preventing heat loss at the time of birth is essential for normal newborn adaptation. Prevent heat loss by:

- Prewarming warmer prior to birth
- Evaluating environment for temperature instability
- Immediately drying infant at time of birth with warmed blankets
- Removing wet blankets
- Placing infant skin-to-skin with mother
- Covering infant with warmed blankets
  - Placing hat on newborn's head
- Initiating early breastfeeding
- Monitoring temperature by axillary temperature assessment
- Placing infant under radiant warmer if low temperature persists
- Assessing blood glucose level; hypoglycemia often precedes cold stress
- Early feeding if hypoglycemia is present
- Placing infants who are unable to maintain body temperature in a prewarmed isolette and transferring them to the high-risk nursery or neonatal intensive care unit
- Delaying initial bath until three normal temperature readings have been obtained

Table 2.1

Types of Heat Loss	
Evaporation	Heat loss occurs from the respiratory tract and skin
Convection	Heat loss to surrounding cooler air
Conduction	Heat loss to solid objects in contact with the body
Radiation	Heat loss to surrounding cooler objects that are not in direct contact with the body

FREQUENCY OF NEWBORN EXAMINATIONS IN FIRST 24 HOURS OF LIFE

Perform the initial newborn examination within 2 hours of birth and a complete nursing assessment when the newborn is admitted to the newborn nursery. Monitor vital signs every 30 minutes for the first 2 hours after birth. Once initial vital signs are completed and are stabilized, vital sign frequency is examined per agency policy but typically during each shift, usually every 8 to 12 hours.

Fast Facts

A physical examination by a practitioner should be performed within the first 24 hours of birth and again prior to discharge.

PROMOTION OF PARENT–INFANT ATTACHMENT

Early positive interactions between the parents and the newborn help to facilitate parent–infant attachment. The nurse can provide the following interventions to aid in the attachment process:

- Place infant skin-to-skin with parent.
- Encourage early breastfeeding.
- Delay newborn assessment and procedures.
- Perform assessment and procedures at the bedside and provide findings to parents.
- Educate parents on normal newborn characteristics and behaviors.
- Advise parents on what to expect in terms of infant behavior and interaction with others.
- Encourage parents to touch newborn.
- Encourage rooming-in and constant contact.
- Assist parents in providing care for the newborn.

- Include siblings and extended family in early interactions with the newborn.
- Encourage eye contact.
- Demonstrate swaddling procedure.
- Encourage parents to rock their infants, hold them upright, and talk to them.
- Describe normal sleep–wake patterns.

APGAR SCORING

The Apgar is a screening test that was developed by Dr. Virginia Apgar in 1952 and is now used worldwide to quickly assess the health of an infant both 1 minute and 5 minutes after birth (Table 2.2). The 1-minute Apgar test measures the newborn's tolerance of the birth, whereas the 5-minute test assesses how well the newborn is adapting to the external environment.

The Apgar score is determined by the following:

- Heart rate
- Breathing
- Activity and muscle tone
- Reflexes
- Skin color

Over 98% of infants have a 5-minute Apgar score of greater than 7. Low 5-minute Apgar scores are not necessarily indicative of long-term adverse health outcomes. Low 5-minute scores are most commonly associated with traumatic births, cesarean births, and fluid in the neonate's lungs. If the score remains below 7 at 5 minutes, a 10-minute Apgar score can be given, with continued testing every 5 minutes until 20 minutes of age. Apgar scores of 7 to 10 at 5 minutes are considered normal.

Fast Facts

Apgar scores lower than 7 indicate ongoing medical intervention is warranted.

GESTATIONAL AGE ASSESSMENT

Gestational age assessment is important for determining needs and possible risks in the early neonatal period. Multiple gestational age

Table 2.2

Apgar Scoring System			
Characteristics	Score of 0	Score of 1	Score of 2
Color	Blue or pale over entire body	Acrocyanosis with pink body	Body pink all over, including extremities
Heart rate	Absent	<100 bpm	>100 bpm
Reflexes	No response to stimulation	Grimace, weak cry with stimulation	Vigorous crying or pulls away with crying
Activity	None	Some flexion	Flexed arms and legs that resist extension
Respiratory	Absent	Weak, irregular gasping	Strong, lusty cry

assessment methods are available to evaluate and determine the newborn's gestational age. These tests evaluate the newborn's appearance, skin texture, motor function, and reflexes. The physical maturity portion of the exam should be performed within the first 2 hours of birth. The neuromuscular maturity examination should be completed within 24 hours after birth. The four factors that are used include muscle tone, joint mobility, automatic reflexes, and fundus exam (Ballard et al., 1991).

The new Ballard score system was developed in 1991 to screen extremely premature infants (starting at 20 gestational weeks) to determine gestational age through neuromuscular and physical assessment (see Exhibit 2.1). New recommendations also address infants that were in breech presentation, since transient flexor fatigue can skew the score. In cases of breech presentation, scores can be adapted from the popliteal angle and heel to ear scores, or the exam can be deferred for 24 to 48 hours when the muscle tone has returned to normal.

PHYSICAL MATURITY CHARACTERISTICS

The newborn's physical characteristics are examined. These include:

- Skin—ranges from sticky and red in preterm infants to smooth or cracking or peeling in postmature infants.
- Lanugo (the soft downy hair on a baby's body)—absent in immature babies, appears with maturity, and then disappears again with postmaturity.
- Plantar creases—these creases on the soles of the feet range from absent to covering the entire foot depending on the maturity.

Exhibit 2.1

New Ballard Score Gestational Age Assessment Chart (1991)

Neuromuscular Maturity

Score	-1	0	1	2	3	4	5
Posture							
Square window (wrist)	>90°	90°	60°	45°	30°	0°	
Arm recoil		180°	140°–180°	110°–140°	90°–110°	<90°	
Popliteal angle	180°	160°	140°	120°	100°	90°	<90°
Scarf sign							
Heel to ear							

Physical Maturity

								Maturity Rating	
Skin	Sticky, friable, transparent	Gelatinous, red, translucent	Smooth, pink; visible veins	Superficial peeling and/or rash; few veins	Cracking, pale areas; rare veins	Parchment, deep cracking; no vessels	Leathery, cracked wrinkled	Score	Weeks
Lanugo	None	Sparse	Abundant	Thinning	Bald areas	Mostly bald		-10	20
Plantar surface	Heel-toe 40-50 mm: -1 <40 mm: -2	>50 mm, no crease	Faint red marks	Anterior transverse crease only	Creases anterior ⅔	Creases over entire sole		-5	22
								0	24
Breast	Imperceptible	Barely perceptible	Flat areola, no bud	Stippled areola, 1–2 mm bud	Raised areola, 3–4 mm bud	Full areola, 5–10 mm bud		5	26
								10	28
Eye/Ear	Lids fused loosely: -1 tightly: -2	Lids open; pinna flat; stays folded	Slightly curved pinna; soft; slow recoil	Well curved pinna; soft but ready recoil	Formed and firm, instant recoil	Thick cartilage, ear stiff		15	30
								20	32
								25	34
Genitals (male)	Scrotum flat, smooth	Scrotum empty, faint rugae	Testes in upper canal, rare rugae	Testes descending, few rugae	Testes down, good rugae	Testes pendulous, deep rugae		30	36
								35	38
								40	40
Genitals (female)	Clitoris prominent, labia flat	Clitoris prominent, small labia minora	Clitoris prominent, enlarging minora	Majora and minora equally prominent	Majora large, minora small	Majora cover clitoris and minora		45	42
								50	44

Source: Used with permission Ballard, J. L., Khoury, J. C., Wedig, K., Wang, L., Eilers-Walsman, B. L., & Lipp, R. (1991). New Ballard score, expanded to include extremely premature infants. *Journal of Pediatrics, 119*, 417–423. doi:10.1016/s0022-3476(05)82056-6

- Breast—the thickness and size of breast tissue and areola (the darkened nipple area) are assessed.
- Eyes and ears—eyes (fused or open) and amount of cartilage and stiffness of the ear tissue are assessed.
- Genitals, male—the presence of testes and appearance of scrotum, from smooth to wrinkled, are assessed.
- Genitals, female—the appearance and size of the clitoris and the labia are assessed.

NEUROMUSCULAR MATURITY CHARACTERISTICS

The neuromuscular characteristics used to determine gestational age include:

Posture	How the baby holds his or her arms and legs
Square window	How much the baby's hand can be flexed toward the wrist
Arm recoil	How much the baby's arms "spring back" to a flexed position
Popliteal angle	How much the baby's knee extends
Scarf sign	How far the elbow can be moved across the baby's chest
Heel to ear	How close the baby's foot can be moved to the ear

References

Ballard, J. L., Khoury, J. C., Wedig, K., Wang, L., Eilers-Walsman, B. L., & Lipp, R. (1991). New Ballard score, expanded to include extremely premature infants. *Journal of Pediatrics, 119*, 417–423. doi:10.1016/s0022-3476 (05)82056-6

Gomella, T., Eyal, F., & Bany-Mohammed, F. (2020). *Gomella's neonatology: Management, procedures, on-call problems, and drugs*. Philadelphia, PA: McGraw-Hill Education.

Hansen, A. R., Eichenwald, E. C., Stakr, A. R., & Martin, C. R. (2016). *Cloherty & Stark's manual of neonatal care* (8th ed.). St. Louis, MO: Lippincott, Williams, & Wilkins.

3

Newborn Procedures

During the early newborn period, a number of procedures should be conducted to ensure the infant is being properly screened and that preventative care practices are being conducted. The nurse conducts multiple procedures during this time period to ensure a smooth transition during the newborn period.

During this part of the orientation, the nurse will be able to:

1. Identify critical procedures that should be performed in the first 24 hours after birth.
2. Ensure that the group streptococcal screening (GBS) status is documented in newborn's chart.
3. Collect and label the laboratory specimens including the recommended uniform screening panel (RUSP), bilirubin level, and cord blood.
4. Facilitate the collection of cord blood and proper labeling of specimens for parents who choose cord blood banking.
5. Perform Vitamin K administration and erythromycin eye prophylaxis administration within 1 hour of birth.
6. Document results of hearing screening with proper identification of newborns who warrant rescreening.

NEWBORN PROCEDURES

The newborn undergoes a number of procedures during the first hours after birth. Nurses should provide new parents with detailed information on the rationale for the procedure, what the procedure involves, and expected outcomes for each procedure. Some parents may have concerns and fears about some procedures and require reassurance and education from the nursing staff.

➡ High Risk Care

Identify neonatal sepsis risk early to prevent serious adverse outcomes. Group streptococcal screening (GBS) is recommended for all pregnant women at 36 weeks. Intravenous administration of penicillin for at least 4 hours prior to birth is recommended (Hansen, Eichenwald, Stakr, & Martin, 2016).

Risk Factors

- Preterm birth prior to 37 completed weeks
- Urinary or gastrointestinal infection with GBS
- Inadequate GBS prophylaxis antibiotic administration prior to birth
- Maternal fever, prolonged rupture of membranes (>18 hours)
- Signs of chorioamnionitis

Routine Laboratory Screenings

Infants of diabetic mothers, small-for-gestational age infants (SGA), large-for-gestational age (LGA) infants, and premature infants should undergo routine screening for abnormal glucose levels. The recommended uniform screening panel (RUSP) is a comprehensive metabolic newborn screening series that is mandated in all 50 states and screens for 32 core conditions and 26 secondary conditions. Screening is recommended 24 to 72 hours after birth and should be performed prior to discharge for infants born in all hospital and birthing facilities. For infants born at home, collection is required within 72 hours of giving birth.

Bilirubin Screening

It is estimated that 85% of newborns develop clinical jaundice. Levels above 12 mg/dL are diagnostic for physiological jaundice. Routine screening for hyperbilirubinemia should include a visual assessment, a review of risk factors for hyperbilirubinemia, and when indicated, a serum bilirubin level and the assignment of a bilirubin risk zone score. A total serum bilirubin measurement can be obtained with routine blood collection of the RUSP.

➡ High Risk Care

Infants with risk factors should have a total serum bilirubin level drawn prior to discharge along with a bilirubin risk value score (Gomella, Eyal, & Bany-Mohammed, 2020).

Risk Factors

- Premature birth
- Hemolytic disease
- G6PD deficiency
- East Asian ethnicity
- Excessive bruising
- Vacuum-assisted birth
- Asphyxia
- Sepsis
- Acidosis
- Albumin levels <3.0 mg/dL
- Presence of a cephalohematoma
- Sibling with a history of the need for phototherapy
- Exclusive breastfeeding with initial weight loss

Bilirubin levels peak at 72 to 96 hours after birth. Levels rising more than 0.2 mg/dL/hour warrant immediate phototherapy. Severe hyperbilirubinemia associated with neurological injury is seen when total bilirubin levels exceed 25 g/dL.

Cord Blood Testing

Cord blood testing is done at the time of birth after the umbilical cord is clamped and cut. When cord blood is drawn, another clamp is placed 8 to 10 inches away from the first. The isolated section is then cut, and a blood sample is collected into a specimen tube. Cord blood testing is not always performed, but can be done for the following testing purposes:

- Bilirubin levels
- Blood culture (if an infection is suspected)
- Blood gases, to evaluate the oxygen, carbon dioxide, and pH levels
- Blood type and Rh
- Complete blood count
- Glucose levels
- Platelet count

Cord Blood Banking

Cord blood banking is an elective procedure in which the parents opt to have the newborn's cord blood collected and stored (autologous) for personal or family use or donated for (allogeneic) public use. Cord blood contains stem cells that can be used to treat more than 80 diseases (Davidson, Ladewig, & London, 2020).

Diseases Treated With Cord Blood

- Leukemias
- Myleodysplastic syndromes
- Lymphomas
- Anemias
- Disorders of blood cell production
- Inherited immune system disorders
- Phagocyte disorders
- Transplants for inherited immune disorders
- Inherited metabolic disorders
- Certain solid tumors
- Neurological, autoimmune, and cardiovascular disorders
- Diabetes
- Genetic and metabolic disorders
- Orthopedic disorders
- Respiratory, reproductive, and ocular diseases
- Wound care

Families with a history of rare disorders, neurological conditions, or cancers may opt to collect cord blood for future use by the child or other family members. Cord blood collection involves a significant cost that is incurred by the family.

Vitamin K Administration

Vitamin K is administered for the prevention of hemorrhage in the first few days of life. Several states have adopted statues mandating administration of vitamin K within 24 hours of birth. Infants who do not receive vitamin K injections are 81 times more likely to develop vitamin K deficiency bleeding (VKDB). Due to the absence of gut flora and low prothrombin levels at birth, newborns are at an increased risk for hemorrhage. Vitamin K_1 (AquaMEPHYTON) is administered via intramuscular injection into the vastus lateralis muscle. The injection is typically given within the first hour after birth. While an oral form of vitamin K is available, treatment with the oral preparation is not found to be as effective and is therefore not routinely recommended.

Fast Facts

Vitamin K injections should always be administered prior to a circumcision procedure due to the risk of bleeding.

Erythromycin Gel Administration to Eyes

Ophthalmia neonatorum (ON) was once a common cause of blindness in newborns in the United States and remains a leading cause of neonatal blindness in developing countries. Prophylactic antibiotic eye treatment is recommended and legally required in some states at the time of birth to prevent the transmission of infection during the birth process. The majority of ON is caused from chlamydia or gonorrhea viruses. Erythromycin gel is the most commonly used agent to prevent infection. The ointment is administered into the lower conjunctival sac of each eye. The ointment may cause edema, blurred vision, and some discomfort that resolves in 1 to 2 days. Eye treatment should be administered within 1 hour of birth.

Hepatitis B Vaccine

Hepatitis B vaccination is now recommended for all newborns at the time of birth. Infants should receive the initial immunization in the hospital and complete the series by the age of 12 to 18 months. Infants weighing less than 2,000 grams whose mothers are negative for hepatitis B maternal surface antigen can delay the vaccine until 1 month of age or receive the vaccine at the time of discharge from the hospital. Infants born to mothers with an unknown status or a positive hepatitis B surface antigen should receive the vaccine within 12 hours of birth regardless of birth weight.

Hearing Screening

Newborn hearing loss is one of the most commonly occurring birth defects and affects 3 out of 1,000 births. Hearing loss can impede speech, language, social, and cognitive development. Currently, 44 states mandate newborn hearing screening measures. It is estimated that 95% of all newborns in the United States are screened prior to hospital discharge. Screening tests include the auditory brainstem response evaluation or the otoacoustic emission measure. Primary intervention strategies that identify newborn hearing loss are estimated to save over $400,000 in lifetime special education costs per child.

Failed Newborn Hearing Screenings

Parents should be counseled that a failed test can occur as a result of excessive noise in the room, excessive newborn movement during the test, and, most commonly, from amniotic fluid accumulation in the ears. If an infant fails the initial test, a second test is performed at least 1 week later. Infants who fail the second test should be referred to a pediatric audiologist for a more definitive screening.

References

Davidson, M. R., Ladewig, P. L., & London, M. L. (2020). *Old's maternal newborn nursing and women's health across the lifespan* (11th ed.). Boston, MA: Pearson Education.

Gomella, T., Eyal, F., & Bany-Mohammed, F. (2020). *Gomella's neonatology: Management, procedures, on-call problems, and drugs*. Philadelphia, PA: McGraw-Hill Education.

Hansen, A. R., Eichenwald, E. C., Stakr, A. R., & Martin, C. R. (2016). *Cloherty & Stark's manual of neonatal care* (8th ed.). St. Louis, MO: Lippincott, Williams, & Wilkins.

II

Comprehensive Newborn Exam

4

Comprehensive Review of History

The comprehensive review of history includes the maternal medical and social history, genetic history, prenatal history, the course of the labor and birth, and the initial newborn transition to extrauterine life. Many components of this review will guide the nurse in identifying risk factors for certain abnormalities that could potentially be identified during the physical examination. Some historical information will prompt further screening or testing in the newborn period.

During this part of the orientation, the nurse will be able to:

1. List the historical information that is pertinent to review prior to performing the newborn examination.
2. Identify pertinent prenatal factors that should be reviewed prior to conducting a newborn exam.
3. Document potential in utero environmental exposures that can lead to adverse neonatal outcomes.
4. Discuss the importance of obtaining genetic information from a historical perspective.
5. Describe the labor, birth historical data, and neonatal information that should be reviewed.

REVIEW OF HISTORICAL DATA

The comprehensive assessment should include the prenatal and birth history, gestational age assessment, and the physical examination. The prenatal and birth history should include the following variables (Davidson, Ladewig, & London, 2020):

Prenatal History

- Initiation of prenatal care and the number of prenatal visits
- Maternal age
- Last menstrual period (normal length of cycles, regular or irregular menses, normal or abnormal length, and quantity of menstrual flow)
- Dates and results of all ultrasound examinations
- Maternal prenatal or medical risk factors
- Laboratory results for routine screenings
- Prenatal testing results
- Well-being of siblings or children living in the same household (lead exposure, viruses, bacterial infections)
- Infectious disease exposure
- Maternal complications during pregnancy
- Medication use during pregnancy

In Utero Environmental Exposures

- Occupational exposures
- Geographic or home exposures
- Exposure to X-rays
- Source of water (tested well, public water supply, other)
- Ingestion of raw or undercooked meats
- Solvents, paints, toxins, radioactive materials, radon
- Exposure to viral or bacterial illnesses
- Proximity to landfill, hazardous waste sites, incinerator
- Nutritional risks such as consumption of high levels of mercury, fluoride, chlorpyrifos (crop contamination), polycarbonate biphenyls (PCBs; fish).
- Toxin exposure via contaminated soil or water supply (lead, arsenic, tetrachlorethylene; PERC), dichlorodiphenyltrichloroethane
- Exposure to bisphenol A (BPA) in beverage containers and plastic containers

Socioeconomic Factors

- Family's place of residence

- Socioeconomic status
- Paternal history
- Presence of the father in the newborn's life
- Exposure to intimate partner violence
- Identification of decision-maker for healthcare decisions
- Cultural influences that impact childrearing and healthcare decision-making
- Other biological children and, if they reside with parents, patterns of abuse or neglect and social services/child protective services involvement
- Immunization status of other children in the household
- Family history of substance abuse
- Legal issues involving parents
- Smoking and exposure to secondhand smoke in the household
- Substance abuse by family members
- Work history of the parents
- Household factors including connected and functioning utilities (running water, heat, and electrical services)
- Crime patterns and neighborhood violence
- Firearms in the household
- Safety precautions in place for other children residing in the household (safety locks, baby gates, medications out of reach of children, etc)

Genetic Factors

A careful review of familial disease and genetic conditions can identify possible genetic conditions present in the newborn. Ideally, parents should have undergone genetic counseling during the prenatal period. Any newborn who has a suspected genetic defect should undergo an evaluation with a genetic specialist and karyotype testing (Gomella, Eyal, & Bany-Mohammed, 2020).

Labor and Birth History

- Length of labor
- Length of rupture of membranes
- Presence of maternal fever
- Presence of nonreassuring fetal status
- Spontaneous or induced labor
- Type of birth (vaginal, cesarean section, operative vaginal birth)
- Length of second stage
- Any birth-related complications (shoulder dystocia, prolonged second stage, nonreassuring fetal status)
- Apgar scores
- Need for resuscitation

Neonatal Factors

- Gestational age
- Measurements (weight, length, head and chest circumference)
- Vital signs at birth and throughout the hospital stay
- Apgar Scores at 1 and 5 minutes (and 10 minutes if performed)
- Documented hypothermia, hypoglycemia, or hyperthermia
- Presence of newborn reflexes indicating a healthy transition
- Type of feeding and feeding patterns
- Urine and stooling patterns
- Symptoms of neonatal abstinence syndrome (jitteriness, abnormal crying, poor suck, or lethargy)
- Any laboratory results obtained since birth

BEHAVIORAL ASSESSMENT

A newborn behavioral assessment scale assesses the newborn's responses to the environment, their neurological abilities, and other capabilities. The scale includes 28 behavioral and 18 reflex items and is designed to assess the baby's capabilities across different developmental areas as well as describe how the baby reacts to the new environment. Components to be measured include (Hansen, Eichenwald, Stakr, & Martin, 2016):

- Habituation
- Orientation to inanimate and animate visual and auditory stimulation
- Motor activity
- Variations in alert states, state changes, and color changes
- Self-quieting abilities
- Social behaviors (cuddling)

Fast Facts

Newborn behaviors vary considerably during the initial 72 hours of birth; therefore, a complete behavioral assessment should not be performed prior to 3 days of life.

NEONATAL ABSTINENCE SCREENING

Neonatal abstinence screening (NAS) is indicated for all infants with potential intrauterine maternal drug exposure. NAS refers to a variety of adverse symptoms that occur in newborn infants who are experiencing withdrawal symptoms (McQueen & Murphy-Owinkton, 2016).

- The incidence of NAS is 55% to 94% of all exposed newborns.
- The severity of symptoms is directly associated with the specific drug used, amount of drug exposure, the last use of the drug, and the newborn's gestational age.
- Initial symptoms may occur within 3 hours of birth (alcohol withdrawal) or as late as 14 days after birth (barbiturate withdrawal).
- Due to physiological differences (reduced body fat and differences in metabolic rates), preterm infants may exhibit fewer symptoms than near-term and term infants.
- Initial laboratory testing may include maternal and neonatal urine drug screens.
- Meconium and umbilical cord blood drug screenings provide a greater window into maternal use.
- Frequent vital signs should be obtained to assess physiological changes in neonatal status.

Screening Tools to Monitor Symptoms of Withdrawal

Each facility may utilize different screening tools and protocols based on evidence-based practice standards. The following protocol illustrates a sample approach using the Lipsitz NAS Screening Tool for the initial assessment followed by the Modified Finnegan Neonatal Abstinence Screening Tool for ongoing assessments (McQueen & Murphy-Owinkton, 2016).

Lipsitz Neonatal Abstinence Screening Tool

- The Lipsitz Tool is a modified briefer tool for initial screening to determine if ongoing screening with the Modified Finnegan NAS Tool is warranted. Some facilities may opt to utilize the Litsitz Screening Tool as their only measure, but this approach is less common (Table 4.1).
- Screening should be performed every 3 hours for the first 72 to 96 hours.
- It is recommended that newborns exposed to narcotics or opioids be screened for the first 72 hours, and those exposed to suboxone or methadone undergo screening for the first 96 hours.
- A score of 4 or higher indicates that pharmacological therapy is warranted.

Table 4.1

Lipsitz Neonatal Abstinence Screening Tool				
Signs	Score of 0	Score of 1	Score of 2	Score of 3
Tremors (muscle movements in limbs)	Normal	Minimal increased when hungry or disturbed	Moderate/marked increased when undisturbed, stops when fed or cuddled	Marked or increased even when undisturbed, going on-to seizure-like movements
Irritability (Excessive Crying)	None	Slightly increased	Slightly increased Moderate to severe irritability when disturbed or hungry	Marked irritability even when undisturbed
Reflexes	Normal	Increased	Markedly increased	
Stools	Normal	Explosive, fewer than 8 per day	Explosive, 8 or more per day	
Muscle tone	Normal	Increased	Rigidity	
Skin abrasions	None	Redness of elbows, heels, pressure points when supine	Breakdown of skin at pressure points	
Respiratory rate (BPM)	<55	55 to 75	76 to 95	
Repetitive Sneezing	No	Yes		
Repetitive Yawning	No	Yes		
Forceful vomiting	No	Yes		
Fever >38°C or 100.4°F	No	Yes		

Modified Finnegan Neonatal Abstinence Screening Tool (Exhibit 4.1)

- This is a scoring tool that measures 21 different indicators that are weighted between 1–5.
- Pharmacological intervention is recommended for newborns scoring >8.
- Scoring should be started at 2 hours after birth and completed every 4 hours during the first 24 hours following birth in newborns with scores less than 8. If scores are >8, monitoring should be conducted every 2 hours. Scoring at 2 hour intervals should continue until a score >7 is present for 24 hours.
- Once a 24 interval of less than 7 occurs, 4-hour intervals should continue for 4 days, providing pharmacological therapy is not being administered.
- During pharmacotherapy, scoring should be performed every 2 hours with scores >8. Once scores are <7 for 24 hours, scoring can be maintained at 4 hour intervals.

Exhibit 4.1

Modified Finnegan Scoring System

System	Signs and Symptoms	Score	AM			PM			Comments
Central Nervous System Disturbances	Excessive high-pitched (or other) cry < 5 mins	2							
	Continuous high-pitched (or other) cry > 5 mins	3							
	Sleeps < 1 hour after feeding	3							
	Sleeps < 2 hour after feeding	2							
	Sleeps < 3 hour after feeding	1							
	Hyperactive Moro reflex	2							
	Markedly hyperactive Moro reflex	3							
	Mild tremors when disturbed	1							
	Moderate-severe tremors when disturbed	2							
	Mild tremors when undisturbed	3							
	Moderate-severe tremors when undisturbed	4							
	Increased muscle tone	1							
	Excoriation (chin, knees, elbow, toes, nose)	1							
	Myoclonic jerks (twitching/jerking of limbs)	3							
	Generalized convulsions	5							
Metabolic Vasomotor Respiratory Disturbances	Sweating	1							
	Hyperthermia 37.2-38.3C	1							
	Hyperthermia > 38.4C	2							
	Frequent yawning (> 3-4 times / scoring interval)	1							
	Mottling	1							
	Nasal stuffiness	1							
	Sneezing (> 3-4 times / scoring interval)	2							
	Nasal flaring	2							
	Respiratory rate > 60/min	1							
	Respiratory rate > 60/min with retractions	2							
Gastrointestinal Disturbances	Excessive sucking	1							
	Poor feeding (infrequent/uncoordinated suck)	2							
	Regurgitation (> 2 times during/post feeding)	2							
	Projectile vomiting	3							
	Loose stools (curds/seedy appearance)	2							
	Watery stools (water ring on nappy around stool)	3							
	Total Score								
	Date/Time								
	Initials of Scorer								

Source: Reproduced with permission from Finnegan, L. P. (1990). Neonatal abstinence syndrome: Assessment and pharmacotherapy. In N. Nelson (Ed.), *Current Therapy in Neonatal—Perinatal Medicine* (2nd ed.). Toronto, ON, Canada: BC Decker.

- Performance of the test should be performed 30–60 minutes after a feeding when the baby is awake. The baby should be awakened to obtain the score, and should be consoled and soothed to avoid active crying.
- If pharmacotherapy has been completed and scores of <8 have been achieved, screening can be discontinued after 3 days.

References

Davidson, M. R., Ladewig, P. L., & London, M. L. (2020). *Old's maternal newborn nursing and women's health across the lifespan* (11th ed.). Boston, MA: Pearson Education.

Gomella, T., Eyal, F., & Bany-Mohammed, F. (2020). *Gomella's neonatology: Management, procedures, on-call problems, and drugs*. Philadelphia, PA: McGraw-Hill Education.

Hansen, A. R., Eichenwald, E. C., Stakr, A. R., & Martin, C. R. (2016). *Cloherty & Stark's manual of neonatal care* (8th ed.). St. Louis, MO: Lippincott, Williams, & Wilkins.

McQueen, K., & Murphy-Owinkton, J. (2016). Neonatal abstinence syndrome. *New England Journal of Medicine, 375*(25), 2468–2479. doi:10.1056/NEJMra1600879

5

Newborn Examination

Each infant undergoes an initial physical examination in the delivery room immediately after birth to detect gross abnormalities and birth defects and to assess the newborn's transition to extrauterine life. A comprehensive examination is then typically performed within the first 2 hours of birth, once the newborn enters the nursery. The nurse performs the initial assessment in the delivery room and then completes the comprehensive examination. The pediatric care provider is then notified of the infant's status. Any abnormalities identified may warrant prompt intervention or referral for additional assessments from specialty providers.

During this part of the orientation, the nurse will be able to:

1. Describe the importance of documenting the initial neonatal weight and measurements.
2. Describe the normal newborn appearance.
3. List the routine measurement data that are obtained during a comprehensive newborn examination.
4. Discuss normal skin variations present in newborn infants.
5. Compare and contrast normal and abnormal physical characteristics in the newborn.

WEIGHT AND MEASUREMENTS

Weight and measurements provide initial data then used throughout infancy to track growth and development. Background information related to weight and measurements includes (Hansen, Eichenwald, Stakr, & Martin, 2016):

- Shortly after birth, the newborn is weighed. In the acute care setting, newborns are typically weighed every 24 hours. Upon discharge, weights and measurements are obtained at each pediatric visit.
- The weight is recorded in both pounds and grams. The average Caucasian infant weighs 3,405 grams (7 pounds 8 ounces). Other races tend to have infants with lower birth weights.
- Infants may lose 10% to 15% of their birth weight during the first few days of life. Exclusively breastfed infants warrant close assessment for weight loss.
- Larger and premature infants often experience greater weight loss. Initial weight loss occurs in the first few days after birth.
- After the first week of life until the age of 6 months, infants typically gain 7 ounces per week. The infant's weight should be plotted on a maturity-and-growth chart.
- Length is obtained by stretching the infant fully and measuring from the top of the head to the heel with the infant in a straightened position.
- The average length for a full-term newborn is 50 cm (20 inches), with a range of 48 to 52 cm (18 to 22 inches).
- Infants typically grow 1 inch per month during the first 6 months of life.
- Head circumference is obtained by measuring the prominent portion of the occiput and extending the tape to above the eyebrows to obtain the circumference of the head.
- The circumference of the head should be 2 cm greater than the chest circumference.
- The average head circumference is 32 to 37 cm (12.5 to 14.5 inches).
- Molding, caput, and cephalohematomas can alter the measurement.
- Reassessing the measurement at 2 days of age often provides a more accurate measurement.
- Chest circumference is measured by placing the measuring tape over the nipple line in the front and at the lower edge of the scapula in the back.

- The average chest circumference is 32 cm (12.5 inches), with a normal range of 30 to 35 cm (12 to 14 inches).
- Abdominal circumference can also be recorded, but, in general, it is not a standardized measurement.

SKIN

Skin variations are common and occur for many reasons:

- Newborns typically have a ruddy complexion due to limited brown fat and increased red blood cells in blood vessels that are close to the surface.
- Dryness, peeling, and cracking can occur and are more common in postdate newborns.
- Skin color varies based on ethnicity.

  - Caucasian newborns are typically pinkish in color immediately after birth.
  - African American newborns range from a pale pink with a yellowish or red hue to a reddish-brown color.
  - Asian and Hispanic babies are typically pink in color, rosy red with a yellow hue, or have an olive or yellow skin tone.

Jaundice can occur within 24 hours of birth. Various skin variations are common in newborns. These variations are found in Table 5.1.

HEAD AND NECK

The newborn may have variations in the head directly associated with the birth process.

- The newborn head is often molded and misshaped due to the birth process.
- *Molding* occurs, allowing the cranial bones to change shape and overlap to facilitate vaginal birth.
- Due to variations in head shape after birth, the head circumference measure may not be accurate during the first few days of life.
- The head may be covered by hair, although some infants are born with no hair at all. In general, any variation in normal hair distribution, texture, or quantity can indicate abnormalities in metabolic, genetic, or abnormalities/disorders.

Table 5.1

Skin Variations in Newborns

Skin Variation	Physical Description	Common Conditions Associated With Skin Condition
Acrocyanosis	Bluish coloration in hands and feet	Common in the first 6 hours after birth. Can also be associated with circulatory issues and cold stress.
Erythema toxicum	Eruption of lesions around hair follicles that consist of yellow or white pustules or papules with an erythematous base. Also known as newborn rash or flea-bite dermatitis.	None. May be an allergic dermatitis related to clothing.
Forceps marks	Reddened areas, commonly over cheeks or jaw, related to difficult forceps birth	Forceps birth
Harlequin sign	A unilateral color change that develops over one side of the body while the other side remains pale. The dramatic color change is temporary and lasts 1–20 minutes. Multiple recurrent episodes are common.	None known
Jaundice	Yellowish skin color related to increases in bilirubin levels	Prematurity, blood incompatibility, forceps or vacuum birth, hematomas, immature liver function, or oxytocin administration during labor. More common in breastfed infants.
Milia	Exposed sebaceous glands resulting in small raised white spots on the face and nose	None
Mottling	Lace-like patterns of dilated blood vessels that occur as a result of fluctuations in circulation	Cold stress, apnea, sepsis, hypothyroidism

(continued)

Table 5.1

Skin Variations in Newborns (*continued*)

Skin Variation	Physical Description	Common Conditions Associated With Skin Condition
Mongolian spots	Macular areas of bluish-black or gray-blue pigmentation found on the lower back and over the buttocks	More common in African American, Hispanic, and Asian infants
Nevus flammeus (port wine stain)	Capillary angioma below the epidermis with dark red to purple area of dense capillaries that does not change over time	Commonly occurs on the face. Can be a sign of Sturge-Weber syndrome and is associated with seizures and visual issues.
Nevus vasculosus (strawberry mark)	Capillary hemangiomas are collections of capillaries in the dermal and subdermal layers that are raised, clearly defined, and fade over time.	None
Telangiectatic nevi (stork-bite marks)	Pale pink or red spots over the eyelids, nose, lower occipital bone, and back of the neck. Usually resolve by 24 months of age.	None
Vernix caseosa	A whitish cheese-like substance that covers the newborn	More abundant in preterm newborns

- The head has two fontanels that are open between the cranial bones, which allows for head growth during infancy and early childhood. The fontanels should be assessed during the newborn exam:

  - The anterior fontanel is diamond-shaped, is 3 to 4 cm long and 2 to 3 cm wide, and is located between the frontal and parietal bones. Closure occurs by 18 months.
  - The posterior fontanel is triangle shaped, is 0.5 to 1 cm long, and is located between the parietal and occipital bones. Closure occurs between 8 and 12 weeks. The neck is short, creased, and symmetrical in appearance.

- The head is inspected for cuts, bruising, instrument injuries, and puncture wounds that can be caused by fetal scalp electrodes.

- Inspection of the sutures and palpation of the suture lines should be performed to rule out craniosynostosis, craniotabs, and deformational plagiocephaly. Overlapping sutures resulting in molding are common, especially in vaginal births or if entrapment in the pelvis occurred necessitating a cesarean birth.
- Swelling can be associated with caput succedaneum, cephalohematoma, or subgaleal hemorrhage.
- The neck contains skin folds, although the back of the neck lacks skin folds.
- The thyroid is in disposition, but should not be visible on inspection. The shoulders and clavicle are symmetrical, straight, and smooth.

FACE, EYES, EARS, NOSE, AND MOUTH

The face, eyes, ears, nose, and mouth should be assessed. The following findings are common:

- The face should be symmetrical with symmetrical movements.
- Asymmetrical movements may indicate facial paralysis.
- The eyes are equally set and parallel to the pinna of the ear.
- The eyes should be checked to ensure equal pupil size, reaction of pupils to light, blink reflex, red retinal reflex, and any presence of eyelid edema, which can occur.
- Subconjunctival hemorrhages can occur and typically resolve in the first month of life.
- Ears should be inspected for patency and pliability of the cartilage. Preauricular skin tags may be present.
- Pinna of the ear should be in the proper position, with the top of the ears parallel to the outer canthus of the eye and normally formed. Low set ears can indicate chromosomal abnormalities, cognitive disabilities, or organ malformation, such as renal agenesis.
- Nose midline
- Nares patent

  - If respiratory difficulties are present, assess to ensure nares are patent.

- Nasal breathing with mouth closed
- Mouth pink with moist mucous membranes
- Mouth symmetrical with the hard and soft palates intact

  - Asymmetry of the mouth can be associated with birth trauma and can indicate nerve damage.

- Gums smooth and pink
- Epstein pearls (glistening white spots) may be present.
- Supplementary teeth (precocious teeth) may be present.
- Tongue is pink in color with a rough texture, protrudes from the mouth, is proportionate in size to the mouth, and movable in all directions
- Gag and swallowing reflexes should be intact.

Fast Facts

Newborns with Down syndrome and other genetic anomalies may have tongues that protrude, with hypotonia being common, giving them an appearance that the tongue is always sticking out. Infants with Down syndrome also have a narrower palate with a higher curve, which may cause breastfeeding difficulties.

CHEST AND LUNGS

The chest and lungs are assessed and normal characteristics or variations are documented:

- The average chest circumference for a newborn is 32.5 cm (12.5 inches), with a range of 30 to 35 cm (12 to 14 inches).
- The chest is wider than it is long and size varies based on gestational weight.
- The sternum is approximately 8 cm long and may appear to protrude slightly.
- The chest should be a cylinder shape and is symmetrical, with pliable ribs and bilateral expansion.
- The lungs should be bilaterally clear to auscultation at rest and with crying.
- The cough reflex develops within 2 to 3 days of birth.

  - Breast enlargement can occur between 3 to 14 days in both male and female newborns and is considered normal. A white discharge can sometimes occur.

Fast Facts

If rales are present, it likely represents normal atelectasis. Intercostal, subcostal, or supraclavicular retractions are indicative of respiratory compromise and warrant additional assessment and intervention.

CARDIOVASCULAR

The cardiovascular system is evaluated by assessing the heart and heart sounds.

- The fetal heart lies horizontally with the left border extending to the left midclavicular line and the apex between the fourth and fifth intercostal space.
- The apical pulse is located at the fourth intercostal space. Sound transmission in a different area can occur with a pneumothorax, dextrocardia, or diaphragmatic hernia.
- Dysrhythmias can be present and warrant immediate comprehensive examination.
- Auscultation for a full minute can detect abnormalities in rate, rhythm, and heart sound intensity. Variations occur related to activity level, crying, sleep state, and body temperature.
- The normal newborn heart rate is 100 to 160 bpm but may be as high as 180 bpm.
- The heart produces a characteristic "lub dub" sound.
- Murmurs that sound like a slur or swishing sound may be present.

  - The majority of murmurs are benign and resolve in the immediate newborn period.
  - Patent ductus arteriosus and patent foramen ovale are the most common auditory murmurs and typically resolve by the third day following birth.
  - Murmurs associated with tachycardia, respiratory distress, and cyanosis require immediate evaluation.

PERIPHERAL VASCULAR

- Peripheral pulses are palpated to determine any abnormalities.

  - Brachial, femoral, and pedal pulses should be assessed and compared bilaterally.

- Pulses should be symmetrical and be equal in nature.
- Abnormalities in peripheral pulses may indicate cardiac defects or hypervolemia and warrant additional assessment.

ABDOMEN

The normal newborn abdominal exam includes an assessment of the abdomen and abdominal organs.

- Abdomen protrudes and is cylinder-shaped.
- Bowel sounds should be present within 1 hour of birth in all four quadrants.
- Abdomen should be soft and nondistended.
- Liver can be palpated 1 to 2 cm below the right costal margin.
- Spleen is palpated in the lateral aspect of the left upper quadrant.
- The lower portion of the kidney is palpable 1 to 2 cm above the level of the umbilicus.

Fast Facts

Kidney palpation may or may not be performed by the nursing staff. If the palpation is part of the newborn exam, it should be assessed within 6 hours of birth, prior to the intestines filling with air, which makes palpation more difficult.

UMBILICAL CORD

The umbilical cord should be assessed as closely as possible to the time of birth because drying distorts the vessels, making assessment more difficult.

- Cord should contain three vessels, two arteries, and one vein.

  - Newborns with a missing umbilical artery have a 25% risk of having additional defects, including cardiac, skeletal, intestinal, or renal problems.

- Umbilical cord must be covered in Wharton's jelly.
- No evidence of bleeding, odor, and drainage should be present.
- No umbilical hernia should be noted.

  - Umbilical hernias occur and are more common in African males and low-birth-weight infants. Umbilical hernias do not typically require intervention and often resolve by 24 months.

GENITALIA AND ANUS

Formation of the genitals occurs in the first trimester. The newborn's genital exam provides data important for the gestational age assessment. The newborn's genitals are inspected and any abnormalities are documented and warrant assessment from a specialist. Ambiguous genitalia is a rare condition where the genitalia is not clearly male or female or there may be characteristics of both sexes.

The female genitalia has the following characteristics:

- Female labia majora, labia minora, and clitoris all develop based on gestational age.

  - Full-term females will have the labia majora covering the labia minora and clitoris.
  - Premature female newborns will have more prominent labia minora with the clitoris clearly visible.

- A hymen tag or vaginal tag is sometimes present.
- Pseudomenstruation is common, which is characterized by a whitish, blood-tinged discharge occurring as a result of withdrawal of maternal hormones.
- Smegma is a white, cheese-like substance that is often present between the labia.

The male genitalia has the following characteristics:

- Urinary meatus at the tip of the penis

  - Hypospadias occurs when the meatus opening is on the vertical surface of the penis.

- The foreskin should be inspected to ensure it can be retracted properly over the penis.

  - *Phimosis* is a condition in which the foreskin will not adequately retract over the penis and often requires surgical intervention.

- The color and position of the testes are dependent on gestational age.

  - Before 36 weeks, the scrotum is small with few rugae, with the testes in the inguinal canal. By term, the entire scrotum is covered with rugae.
  - At term, a testicle should be palpable in each scrotal sac.

- Each testicle should be palpated separately to confirm it has descended.

  - *Cryptorchidism* is the failure of a testicle to descend and warrants follow-up to prevent long-term complications.

- Hydrocele, which is a collection of fluid in the scrotum, may occur after birth and typically resolves without intervention.

EXTREMITIES

An assessment of the extremities is performed and documented:

- Extremities are inspected and should be symmetrical in size and proportion.
- Arms should be flexible without gross abnormalities, extra digits, webbing, or clubfoot.
- Range-of-motion abnormalities or lack of movement may occur with brachial plexus (partial or complete paralysis of arm related to birth trauma).
- Erb's palsy typically results in upper arm paralysis, in which the arm lies in a limp position and remains motionless.
- Arms should be symmetrical and bend easily with a good range of motion.
- Hands should be inspected and the pattern of palmar creases should be documented.

    - A single palmar crease may be indicative of genetic anomalies and may warrant further testing.

- Legs and feet should be bilaterally symmetrical, with the skin folds of the thighs in equal proportion to each other.
- The Barlow maneuver should be performed to detect congenital hip dysplasia.
- Feet are inspected to ensure they are in a proper position.
- Observe for the presence of clubfoot.
- Positional clubfeet are sometimes present and are most commonly associated with breech position.
- Positional clubfoot is treated with range-of-motion exercises, whereas a true clubfoot will require surgical intervention.

Fast Facts

To assess for hip dysplasia, grasp both thighs simultaneously and adduct the thighs, applying gentle pressure in a downward motion. If the femoral head slips out of the acetabulum, dislocation is probable.

Perform the Ortolani's maneuver when the infant is at rest, with the knees and thighs flexed at a 90-degree angle. Grasp the thigh with the middle finger over the trochanter and lift the thigh toward the acetabulum. With gentle abduction, return the head to the acetabulum and listen for an audible click if the hip is dislocated.

BACK

The back should be inspected:

- Skin is intact over the entire spine.
- Spine should be straight.
- The base of the spine should be carefully evaluated to ensure a nevus pilosus (hairy nevus) is not present.

  - The presence of a nevus pilosus can be associated with spina bifida.

- Some infants may have a pilonidal dimple, which can also be related to spina bifida and warrant further assessment.

Reference

Hansen, A. R., Eichenwald, E. C., Stakr, A. R., & Martin, C. R. (2016). *Cloherty & Stark's manual of neonatal care* (8th ed.). St. Louis, MO: Lippincott, Williams, & Wilkins.

III

Newborn Nutrition

6

Nutritional Needs of the Newborn

Adequate newborn nutrition is essential for human life, and the process of infant feeding is linked with the formation of lasting attachment with the caregiver and stimulates psychosocial development. Parents need extensive education in the basics of newborn feeding to ensure adequate growth during the infancy period. Proper fluid and electrolyte management is essential to prevent dehydration. Dehydration is more common in the newborn period and can either be associated with inadequate fluid intake or dehydration that can occur with increased fluid loss. Hypoglycemia is the most common of glucose instability in the newborn period. Prompt identification and treatment of hypoglycemia in the newborn period is essential.

During this part of the orientation, the nurse will be able to:

1. Identify the nutritional components, including vitamins and minerals, that are essential for normal growth and development in the newborn and infant.
2. Discuss the importance of fluid and electrolyte balance in the newborn period.
3. Identify potential causes of dehydration in the newborn period.
4. Discuss risk factors for hypoglycemia in the newborn.
5. List adverse outcomes associated with hypoglycemia.

NUTRITIONAL NEEDS OF NEWBORNS

In the first few months of life, the brain grows at a rapid rate, and adequate food and nutrition are needed for both physiological and psychological growth and development.

Calories

- For the infant to maintain himself or herself and ultimately grow, the caloric needs for the newborn up to 2 months of age are approximately 110 to 120 calories per kilogram of body weight (50 to 55 kcal/pound) every 24 hours (Table 6.1).
- Calorie needs will vary depending on activity level and growth rate.
- Commercial formulas simulate breast milk and get 9% to 12% of calories from protein and 45% to 55% of calories from lactose carbohydrate. The balance of the formula consists of fat, of which about 10% (4% of the calories) consists of linoleic acid.

Fast Facts

An infant who cries frequently and squirms constantly needs more calories.

Protein

Protein is necessary for the formation of new cells. The newborn requires around 2.2 g/kg of body weight in protein intake daily.

Table 6.1

Energy Expenditure of an Infant	
Resting energy use	40 kcal/kg/day
Minimal activity	2–4 kcal/kg/day
Occasional cold stress	10 kcal/kg/day
Loss of energy from bowel movements	10 kcal/kg/day
Growth	40 kcal/kg/day
Total	100–105 kcal/kg/day

Unaltered cow's milk is not recommended for newborns because 16% of its calories contain protein, whereas human milk contains 8%; the protein in cow's milk can be overwhelming to the newborn's kidneys. Additionally, cow's milk is difficult for the newborn to digest.

Fat

Linoleic acid, an essential fatty acid, is necessary for growth and skin integrity in infants and is found in both breast milk and commercial formulas.

Carbohydrate

Lactose is the most easily digested carbohydrate. Carbohydrates allow protein to be used for building new cells. Additionally, carbohydrates encourage normal water balance and prevent abnormal metabolism of fat. They have been shown to also aid in calcium absorption and improve nitrogen retention.

Fluid

- Neonates are born with an excess of total body water; this is primarily extracellular fluid (ECF).
- Term neonates usually lose between 5% and 10% of their birth weight in the first week of life, and almost all of this weight loss is the excess ECF.
- With a high metabolic rate and immature kidney function that does not fully concentrate urine, the newborn needs to be monitored closely for fluid volume depletion and dehydration.
- Fluid requirements for the newborn are between 150 and 200 mL/kg per 24 hours and should be completely supplied by breastfeeding or formula feeding.

Fast Facts

Term neonate bodies are 75% water, 40% ECF, and 35% intracellular fluid.

Calcium

Calcium is essential for the infant's bone growth. If a newborn's ability to suck is adequate, and the child is receiving the necessary nutrition, a low calcium level seldom occurs.

Iron

Term infants of a mother who had adequate iron intake during pregnancy will be born with iron stores lasting for 3 months, which is when the newborn begins to produce hemoglobin. Most mothers do not get adequate iron in their diet and therefore a supplement is recommended for breast-fed infants for 1 year. Most commercially prepared formulas have iron supplementation for this reason.

Fluoride

Teeth grow into their primary form during pregnancy, so mothers should drink fluoridated water during and after pregnancy to supply the baby. Fluoride is also contained in most commercially prepared formulas. A fluoride supplement of 0.25 mg/day may be given to infants starting at 6 months of age. However, this can be detrimental or stain teeth.

Vitamins

Vitamins are not routinely needed or necessary for bottle-fed infants because vitamins A, C, and D are available to the infant in commercial formulas (Table 6.2). The nutritional needs are based on the gestational age of the neonate. Preterm infants have fewer nutritional daily needs than term infants. Commercial formulas are required to have the minimum recommended dietary reference ranges. Vitamins are naturally found in breast milk; however, breastfed newborns should receive a vitamin D 400 IU per day (or the mother can take 400 IU daily). Vitamins are not routinely given to infants younger than 6 months of age.

Preterm infants have varying vitamin supplementation recommendations. Preterm breastfeeding infants who weigh >2,000 grams and reach 35 corrected gestational weeks should be supplemented with a 1 mL pediatric multivitamin (without iron) daily and ferrous sulfate 10 mg/mL daily. Formula-fed premature infants.

➡ High Risk Care: Fluid and Electrolyte Management

In utero, the fetus's water and electrolyte balance is performed by the placenta. Fluid and electrolyte balance is essential for newborns. The ability to maintain adequate balance can be impaired in the newborn period due to the increased surface-area-to-mass ratio in infants and the reduced kidney absorption capabilities. Newborns

Table 6.2

Vitamin	Term Infant Needs >2,500 g	Preterm Needs <2,500 g	Human Milk (Term and >21 days in Women With Preterm Births) Based on 150 mL/kg/day
A (ug)	700	280	240
D (IU)	400	160	2
E (mg)	7	2.8	0.9
K (ug)	200	80	0.4
Thiamine (mg)	1.2	0.48	30
Riboflavin (mg)	1.4	0.56	75
Niacin (mg)	17	6.8	0.6
Pantothenate (mg)	5	2	0.34
Pyridoxine (mg)	1	0.4	
Biotin (ug)	20	8	1.1
Vitamin B$_{12}$ (ug)	1	0.4	0.11
Ascorbic acid (mg)	80	32	
Folic acid (ug)	140	56	16.5

require, on average, 140–160 mL/kg/day daily fluid. Dehydration is more common in the newborn period and can either be associated with inadequate fluid intake or dehydration that can occur with increased fluid loss. Potential sources of fluid loss for the term newborn include vomiting and dehydration.

Symptoms of Dehydration
- Rapid, weak pulse
- Elevated temperature
- Concentrated, dark urine
- Dry, hard stools
- Specific gravity >1.020
- Depressed fontanelles
- Poor skin turgor

Very preterm and preterm infants have a higher percentage of extracellular fluid. Very-low-birth-weight (VLBW) infants must lose a greater proportion of birth weight to maintain the ECF proportions of term infants. Preterm infants are more likely to experience immature sodium and water loss imbalances from immature renal functioning and interventional or factors related to prematurity including:

- Skin breakdown
- Radiant warmer use
- Phototherapy
- Respiratory water loss
- Inadequate humidification during intubation
- Loose stools
- Ostomy drainage
- Cerebral spinal fluid loss from procedures
- Nasogastric tube or thoracotomy tube drainage

Glucose Stabilization

Hypoglycemia is the most common of glucose instability in the newborn period. Hypoglycemia can affect as many as 54% of newborns (Davidson, Ladewig, & London, 2020).

Risk Factors for Low Blood Glucose Levels

- Large for gestational age (LGA)
- Small for gestational age (SGA)
- Infants of diabetic mothers (IDM)
- Prematurity
- Later preterm gestational age
- Low birth weight (LBW)
- Carbohydrate deficits
- Endocrine deficiency
- Amino acid metabolism defects

Infants who have experienced perinatal stressors, such as sepsis, shock, asphyxia, respiratory depression, hypothermia, and those who received resuscitation at the time of birth are at an increased risk for hypoglycemia. Many infants with hypoglycemia are asymptomatic.

Symptoms of hypoglycemia

- Irritability
- Jitteriness
- Tremors
- Lethargy
- High-pitched cry
- Cyanosis

- Apnea
- Exaggerated Moro reflex
- Seizures
- Low tone
- Difficulty feeding

Table 6.3

Treatment Recommendations for Hypoglycemia in the Newborn				
Initial & Follow-Up Assessment Recommendations	Findings	Interventions	Follow-Up Assessment	Interventions
Asymptomatic newborn within 4 hours of birth	≤25 mg/dL	Breastfeeding or formula feeding	Reassess blood glucose level.	If newborn is unable to tolerate oral feedings, has persistent hypoglycemia, or is unable to maintain normal glucose levels, consider 40% dextrose gel IV glucose.
Second glucose check after feeding or glucose supplementation	≤25 mg/dL	IV glucose and admission to NICU		
Second glucose check after feeding or glucose supplementation	25–40 mg/dL	Breastfeeding or formula feeding	Reassess glucose level 1 hour later.	If <35 mg/dL, IV glucose is warranted.
4–24 hours after birth	<35 dl/dL	Breastfeeding or formula feeding	Reassess glucose level in 1 hour.	If <35 mg/dL, administer glucose.
Second check after initial feeding	35–45 mg/dL	Breastfeeding or formula feeding indicated again	If glucose levels >45 mg/dL, target range has been reached.	Feed every 203 hours.

The screening criteria and interventions suggested are based on the neonate's age (in hours since birth), observance of symptoms, and the plasma glucose levels. Glucose stability should occur within 48 to 72 hours of life and should be >60 mg/dL. Reagent strips are within 10 to 15 mg/dL; thus, if a neonate is experiencing symptoms with borderline glucose levels, a blood glucose level should be obtained. If plasma levels remain abnormal, treatment should be initiated. Treatment guidelines are based on blood glucose values (Table 6.3).

Fast Facts

Plasma glucose levels, which are typically obtained at the bedside, are approximately 15% higher than blood glucose serum levels.

Reference

Davidson, M. R. Ladewig, P. L., & London, M. L. (2020). *Old's maternal newborn nursing and women's health across the lifespan* (11th ed.). Boston, MA: Pearson Education.

7

Breastfeeding

Infant feeding practice decisions involve a variety of factors, including comfort with breastfeeding, modesty, family values, and cultural norms. Some women will not feel comfortable breastfeeding and will choose formula feeding. These women should be fully supported in their decision-making and should receive educational information on proper formula preparation and storage. Premature infants require special attention and may warrant supplemental feedings. Prematurity and low birth weight put some infants at risk for poor postnatal growth in the newborn and early-infancy period. Family education should include variations in growth patterns for families with premature infants.

During this part of the orientation, the nurse will be able to:

1. Name nursing interventions that help support successful breast-feeding in the early postpartum period.
2. List the benefits of breastfeeding.
3. Discuss challenges associated with breastfeeding in the NICU.
4. Identify the contraindications for breastfeeding.
5. Identify proper pumping and storage guidelines for breast milk.
6. Review the discharge preparation for infant feeding instructional information.

BREASTFEEDING

Breastfeeding is the preferred feeding method for the newborn and the ideal nutrition source for infants during the first year of life and beyond. Evidence shows breastfeeding has immediate as well as long-term health benefits.

NURSING INTERVENTIONS TO SUPPORT BREASTFEEDING

Nurses play a major role in educating new parents about the benefits and management of breastfeeding. Key interventions include:

- Helping to initiate breastfeeding within 30 minutes of birth
- Assisting the new mother with breastfeeding and ensuring lactation, even if the infant must be separated from the mother
- Advocating against supplemental feedings other than breast milk unless medically indicated
- Avoiding providing pacifiers to breastfeeding infants until breastfeeding has been well established
- Advocating for mother/infant rooming-in
- Encouraging breastfeeding on demand
- Fostering the establishment of breastfeeding support groups and referring mothers to lactation consultants as needed

PHYSIOLOGY OF BREAST MILK PRODUCTION

Breast milk production occurs in the maternal breasts and relies on hormonal responses for adequate milk production.

- Formed in the acinar or alveolar cells of the mammary glands, breast milk begins to secrete in the fourth month of pregnancy.
- With delivery of the placenta, progesterone levels fall dramatically, which stimulates the production of prolactin (released from the anterior pituitary gland).

- Prolactin stimulates the production of milk.
- Initiation of newborn feeding as soon as possible after birth will start production of prolactin-releasing factor in the hypothalamus.
- Colostrum is a thin, watery, yellow fluid that contains protein, sugar, fat, water, minerals, vitamins, and maternal antibodies, and is produced for the first 3 to 4 days after birth.
- Transitional milk begins to form on days 2 to 4 and may be present up to 10 to 14 days after birth. It is characterized by a creamy milk, and is often referred to by mothers as "their milk coming in."
- As the baby latches on and begins to breastfeed steadily, many mothers begin to notice a tingly pins-and-needles sensation, which indicates that that the milk let-down reflex has occurred.

  - This reflex causes milk to be pushed out of the milk-producing cells into milk ducts so that it is available for feeding. The let-down reflex can be stimulated by the baby's suckling, the approach of feeding time, or just the sound of a baby crying.

- In most women, mature milk begins to appear near the end of the second week after childbirth.
- Mature milk is the final milk that is produced and is composed of 90% water, which is necessary to maintain infant hydration. The other 10% is composed of carbohydrates, proteins, and fats, which are necessary for both growth and energy.

  - There are two types of mature milk: foremilk and hindmilk. Ingestion of both foremilk and hindmilk is necessary to ensure the baby is receiving adequate nutrition.

    - Foremilk: This type of milk is ingested during the beginning of the feeding and contains water, vitamins, and protein.
    - Hindmilk: This type of milk is produced after the initial release of milk and contains higher levels of fat, which is necessary for weight gain.

Fast Facts

During the let-down reflex, the infant's suckling releases oxytocin from the posterior pituitary, which causes the collecting sinuses of the mammary glands to contract, forcing milk forward through the nipples.

Maternal Advantages of Breastfeeding

- Protective function against breast cancer
- Release of oxytocin aids in uterine involution
- Empowering effect
- Reduces cost of feeding
- Promotes optimal maternal–infant attachment

Infant Advantages of Breastfeeding

- Immunoglobulin A (IgA)—binds with large molecules of foreign proteins, including viruses and bacteria
- Lactoferrin—iron-binding protein that interferes with growth of pathogenic bacteria
- Lysozyme—destroys bacteria by dissolving cell membranes
- Bifidus factor—growth-promoting factor for lactobacillus bifidus, which interferes with colonization of bacteria in the gastrointestinal tract, reducing diarrhea
- Ideal electrolyte and mineral composition
- High in lactose, which easily digests sugar (rapid brain growth)
- Protein, nitrogen, and linoleic acid
- Less sodium, potassium, calcium, and phosphorus than formula
- Less potential for allergy development
- Better dental arch

Contraindications for Breastfeeding

- In the United States, mothers who are infected with HIV
- Infants who cannot digest lactose (galactose 1-phosphate uridyltransferase deficiency)
- Herpes lesions on nipples
- Mother on restricted-nutrient diet that prevents quality milk production
- Mother on medications that are inappropriate for breastfeeding
- Mother exposed to radioactive compounds
- Breast cancer

Women with postpartum psychosis or those with a previous episode of postpartum psychosis should be discouraged from breastfeeding. While some medications, even anti-psychotics, can be safely used during lactation, the interference with the sleep cycle is known to be a prepsychotic indicator with women who go on to develop postpartum psychosis. Women should be counseled that, even with protected sleep, the body's natural milk production often results in sleep disturbances (Davidson, Sampson, & Davidson, 2017).

Disadvantages of Breastfeeding

- May transfer microorganisms—Hepatitis B virus, cytomegalovirus, HIV, illicit and prescription drugs, tobacco, or environmental contaminants are ingested by the newborn via breast milk.

PROLONGED JAUNDICE IN BREASTFEEDING INFANTS

Jaundice in breastfeeding infants is caused by pregnanediol, a breakdown product of progesterone found in breast milk. Pregnanediol depresses the action of glucuronyl transferase, the enzyme that converts indirect bilirubin to its direct form, which is excreted in bile. To avoid jaundice in their newborns, women should feed frequently in the immediate birth period because colostrum is a natural laxative that helps the newborn to pass meconium and bile. Pregnanediol remains for 24 to 48 hours.

BREASTFEEDING IN THE NICU (HRC)

The ability to tolerate oral feedings depends on an ability to coordinate sucking, swallowing, and breathing, which is often difficult for premature and medically fragile newborns. Lack of adequate coordination can result in apnea, bradycardia, oxygen desaturation, and aspiration. Premature neonates may have physical alterations that interfere with oral feedings. These factors can impact the neonate's ability to form an adequate seal and vacuum to facilitate breastfeeding.

Physical Alterations That Interfere With Oral Feedings

- Hypotonia
- Immature neurological and gastrointestinal systems
- Medical complications

  - Orofacial abnormalities
  - Gastroesophageal reflux
  - Respiratory compromise

In preterm infants and infants with medical complications, breastfeeding may not be initially possible. The need to provide education, encouragement, and support is imperative. The following factors should be utilized to support early breastfeeding:

- Provide lactation consultation as early as possible after birth.
- Begin pumping every 2 to 3 hours in the immediate postpartum period while awake and every 3 to 4 hours at night.

- Encourage rooming-in (where available in NICU settings) and pumping in close proximity to the infant.
- Infants can be held against the breast to encourage familiarity and support the emotional needs of the mother while they are being given tube feedings.
- Electric pumps should be encouraged. Rental of pumps from the facility of a local facility should be obtained as soon as possible.
- Put the baby to breast as soon as possible. Direct breastfeeding at least once per day in the NICU is associated with breastfeeding at the time of discharge and at 4 months of age (Wambach & Spenser, 2019).
- Healthcare professionals providing interventions and education are associated with a higher incidence of breastfeeding at the time of discharge.

PUMPING AND MILK STORAGE FOR NICU INFANTS (HRC)

Pumping and storage of milk is essential for breastfeeding success for newborns hospitalized in the NICU setting. Very premature infants and those with medical complications may have an extended stay in the NICU setting. Even when mothers room-in, most need to pump and prepare milk for storage during their infant's stay.

Infection control is a primary concern in the NICU setting, so evidence-based practices to minimize the risk of contamination are essential. Education should focus on ensuring the mother is collecting milk to minimize infection risks. These educational guidelines include:

- Wash hands with warm, soapy water (remove jewelry), use disposable paper towels to turn off faucets, and dry hands completely prior to pumping.
- Keep nails trimmed to a short length; artificial nails are a breeding ground for bacteria and should be avoided.
- If a personal pump is being used, clean the pump according to manufacturer's guidelines after each use.
- Clean the surface where the pump is located with disinfectant cleaners or wipes.
- Shared pumps require sterilization in accordance with hospital policies between users in addition to proper cleaning of the surface or area where the pump is located.
- Pump parts should be rinsed with cold water to remove milk residue and then washed in warm, soapy water. Place pump parts on a clean surface to air dry or dry with a clean cloth that does not leave lint residue.

- Label all milk with the mother's name, baby's identifying information (such as bar code labels), date and time of expression, and volume of milk. Single-use containers are ideal, but reusable containers that are properly and thoroughly cleaned in accordance with hospital policies are also acceptable.
- Use preprinted labels whenever possible to reduce the risk of mislabeling. It is preferred that all milk entering the facility be labeled prior to entry to decrease the risk of improper identification.
- Use the "four eyes" principle to ensure that the proper milk is given to the proper infant. This ensures two nurses have double-checked the label and prevents mishandling and/or the incorrect milk from being given to the wrong infant.
- Refrigerate pumped breastmilk or freeze as soon as possible after pumping if it will not be fed to the infant within 4 hours.
- When transporting milk to the facility, use ice packs and an insulated bag to preserve the milk.
- Milk should be used as soon as possible, by the date of oldest milk first.
- Warmed milk is associated with better body temperature regulation in preterm and high-risk infants. Facilities may vary

Table 7.1

Proper Storage of Milk Products			
Type of Milk Product	Safety Duration at Room Temperature	Storage Duration	Freezing Instructions
Expressed breast milk	4 hours	4 days if refrigerated, 3 months if frozen	When thawed to room temperature, use within 4 hours. When thawed in the refrigerator, use within 24 hours.
Fortified breast milk	Not recommended	Refrigerate immediately and use within 24 hours.	Not recommended
Pasteurized donor breast milk	Not recommended	Refrigerate immediately and use within 24 hours.	Not recommended
Reconstituted commercial formula	1 hour	24 hours	Not recommended

in warming practices. Dry warmers have reduced the incidence of infection that can occur when contaminated water enters the breastmilk.

Table 7.1 outlines the proper storage periods for milk products. Proper storage guidelines ensure milk products are safe for infant consumption and reduce the risk of contamination. Because fortification can change the bacterial growth factors, recommendations vary when fortifiers are added to breast milk.

DISCHARGE PLANNING RELATED TO INFANT FEEDING

Optimal growth for neonates and infants requires careful thought about nutrition. Interventions (or lack of them) may have long-term consequences, so discharge teaching is imperative:

- Teach about infant nutrition and answer questions parents may have related to feedings.
- Advise parents that after the first week of life newborns should have 6 to 8 wet diapers/day if achieving adequate fluid intake.

References

Davidson, M. R., Sampson, M., & Davidson, N. S. (2017). Identifying prodromal symptomology in women who have experienced postpartum psychosis: A grounded research study. *International Journal of Pregnancy and Childbirth, 2*(6), 159–165. doi:10.15406/ipcb.2017.02.00041

Wambach, K., & Spenser, B. (2019). *Breastfeeding and human lactation.* Boston, MA: Jones & Bartlett.

8

Common Physiological Breastfeeding Symptoms

It is not uncommon for mothers to experience breastfeeding difficulties in the newborn period. Preparation for breastfeeding can help reduce common difficulties many new mothers may experience. Nurses can provide education in the prevention, identification, and treatment of common breastfeeding issues. Early intervention and assistance with common difficulties helps to ensure the continuation of breastfeeding in the newborn period.

During this part of the orientation, the nurse will be able to:

1. Discuss common educational advice that should be given to mothers during pregnancy to prepare for breastfeeding.
2. Identify the most common issue that interferes with proper latch-on in the newborn period.
3. Detail the importance of changing positions during feedings.
4. Describe interventions to increase a mother's milk supply.
5. Name common symptoms that occur with mastitis.

PREPARATION FOR BREASTFEEDING

- Because breastfeeding is both a natural and a learned process, discussion and education should begin during pregnancy.

- Breastfeeding should begin as soon after birth as possible, and the labor and delivery nurse or birth attendant should be available to assist the mother in proper latching.
- For an adequate latch, it is important that the newborn open his or her mouth wide enough to grasp the nipple and areola when sucking.
- Assistance from a lactation consultant should be initiated for mothers who are struggling with early feedings.

COMMON BREASTFEEDING ISSUES

Many breastfeeding issues occur in the early postpartum period. Nurses and lactation consultants play a vital role in providing support and ensuring proper latch-on and positioning as a means to prevent and treat common breastfeeding issues (Wambach & Spenser, 2019). Table 8.1 outlines common issues that occur, the etiology of the issue, preventive strategies to prevent the issue, along with the symptoms and treatment for each issue.

Fast Facts

Lactation consultants can provide both education and hands-on assistance to new mothers in the early newborn period to reduce the incidence of breastfeeding problems.

Table 8.1

Common Physiological Breastfeeding Symptoms

Breastfeeding Issue	Physiological Etiology	Prevention	Symptoms	Treatment
Engorgement	Vascular and lymphatic congestion that arises from increased blood and lymph supply to the breast. Represents a transient/ temporary problem (lasts approximately 24 hours).	Wearing a well-fitting, supportive bra. Using a breast pump after feeding to completely empty the breast. Using a breast pump after feeding to completely empty the breast.	Breast distention, swelling, hardness, tenderness, and heat. The areola may be too hard for the baby to latch on to.	Standing under the shower and massaging the breast to soften it so the infant can latch on more easily. Applying warm packs for 20 minutes prior to feeding.
Nipple soreness	Pain, irritation, or soreness of the nipple. Strong sucking action of the infant. Sucking too long after the breast is emptied or from the improper positioning. An inappropriate release of the infant from the breast.	Positioning the baby slightly differently for each feeding to avoid pressure on the same area of the areola. Changing feeding positions often (football hold, side-lying, cradle hold).	Pain or soreness, especially noticeable at the time of feeding.	Begin feeding on the side with the least amount of discomfort. Express colostrum or breast milk after nursing and rub into the nipple. Exposing nipples to air for 10 to 15 minutes after feeding. Applying modified lanolin in very small amounts to promote a moisture barrier and healing without scab formation. Avoiding use of a hand pump and educating mother on manual expression.

(continued)

Table 8.1

Common Physiological Breastfeeding Symptoms (continued)

Breastfeeding Issue	Physiological Etiology	Prevention	Symptoms	Treatment
Cracked nipples	Cracks or fissures that appear on the nipple typically associated with improper latch-on or improper positioning. Prolonged cracking beyond the first few weeks can be associated with an infection such as monilia or a bacterial infection.	Ensure that the baby is properly positioned and latched on with each feeding. Proper alignment with the ear, shoulder, hip, and legs symmetrically aligned can prevent pulling and poor latch-on.	Cracks or fissures on nipple. Bleeding may occur.	If baby is improperly latched, break the suck by inserting your finger in a J hook position to break the seal of the latch. Relatch infant ensuring the chin latched on as much as the areola as possible and comes over the top of the nipple. If slipping occurs, break seal and reattach. If cracking continues and infant is unable to latch, the infant should be assessed for a shortened frenulum.
Inadequate milk supply	Inadequate milk supply results from not completely emptying the breast with regular and complete feedings. Milk forms in response to being used. If completely emptied, milk production will refill the breast completely and establish a regular supply.	Feed infant at least every 2–3 hours with no longer than a 4-hour interval once per day. Completely empty breast with each feeding.	Infant crying between feedings, unable to satisfy infant, infant fails to fall asleep during or after feeding. Mother may report a sensation that the breasts fail to feel full.	If half emptied, the breast will refill halfway, and milk production will be insufficient. New mothers need to feed every 2–3 hours for about 10–15 minutes on each breast. If infant falls asleep during feeding, infant should be awakened and encouraged to eat longer. Bottles should not be offered until 6 weeks of age or when breastfeeding has been well established.

Plugged ducts	A plugged duct occurs when the milk duct within the breast is obstructed between the breast and the nipple itself, resulting in a tender lump.	An area with redness, warmth, and tenderness on one breast that may increase gradually in size. Skin may be red or pink in color. A white bump sometimes forms on the nipple itself. May result in pain in the breast or shooting pains in the nipple.	Frequent feedings (every 2–3 hours), starting with the affected side first. Use warm compresses or a warm shower or bath with gentle massage prior to feeding. Use massage after feeding to attempt to drain milk from affected area. Use of breast pump or manual expression to drain milk is recommended after feedings.
	Routine feedings every 2–3 hours using varying feeding positions allow for different areas of drainage within the breast tissue , thus decreasing the incidence of plugged ducts. Infants should be fed 8–12 feedings per day or when signs of hunger are observed. Avoid tight-fitting bras.		
Mastitis	Inflammation of the breast typically caused by an infectious process that most commonly occurs during the first 2 months of breastfeeding. Bacteria often enters nipple when a portal of entry, such as a cracked nipple, is present. Also known as *lactational mastitis*. Most common pathogen is *Staphylococcus aureus*; less common organisms are *Streptococcus* or *Escherichia coli*.	Painful, red, tender area. Warm to touch. Malaise or flu-like symptoms. May have a sudden onset. Fever, chills, and body aches often occur.	Antibiotics are indicated. Dicloxacillin 125–500 mg QID for 5–14 days. Give medication 1 hour before meal or 2 hours after meal. Flucloxacillin 500 mg QID can also be given. If an allergy to penicillin exists, use cephalexin. Women with severe penicillin allergies or an immediate allergy should be treated with clindamycin or erythromycin. Frequent breast emptying is necessary. Apply heat and massage to remove lump and open plugged ducts. Warm and hot compresses TID will help release buildup of milk in the ducts. *Women should receive education that milk is not infected and ongoing nursing should be encouraged.*
	Frequent feedings, (every 2–3 hours) in the newborn period and every 4–6 hours in older infants. Avoid engorgement and skipped feedings of pumping sessions. Varying feeding position helps ensure all milk ducts are emptied. More common in cracked or sore nipples. Proper-fitting nursing bras help prevent plugged ducts, which can lead to mastitis.		

(continued)

Chapter **8** Common Physiological Breastfeeding Symptoms

Table 8.1

Common Physiological Breastfeeding Symptoms (continued)

Breast abscess	Painful area of tissue that becomes infected and forms a pocket of mucopurulent pus within the breast. Typically occurs as a result of untreated, late treatment, or improper treatment of mastitis. Women with diabetes, long-term steroid treatments, heavy smokers, and previous breast surgeries are at greater risk.	Prompt treatment of plugged ducts. if unable to successfully treat a plugged duct, consultation with a lactation consultant or healthcare professional is indicated. Prompt treatment of mastitis can prevent an abscess.	Painful, red, hot-to-touch, hard, unilateral mass occurs. Breast becomes swollen and engorged. Purulent exudate from the nipple may occur. Mass does not resolve with antibiotic treatment. High fever and flu-like symptoms may occur.	Needle aspiration with antibiotic treatment based on sensitivities if less than 3 cm. Masses greater than 3 cm require surgical removal and are drained via catheter and left open to heal. Deep masses may require removal under general anesthesia. Packing of the wound is usually required.

References

Wambach, K., & Spenser, B. (2019). *Breastfeeding and human lactation.* Boston, MA: Jones & Bartlett.

9

Formula and Feeding Infants With Special Needs

Infants may receive breastmilk, formula, specialty formulas, or a combination of both formula and breastmilk. Effective feeding techniques are important to ensure the infant is getting optimal intake. Premature infants may require specialty formula, tube feedings, or feeding support in the early newborn period. Infants with anatomical issues may require specialized bottles or feeding support. Postnatal growth is an important indicator of newborn feeding adequacy.

During this part of the orientation, the nurse will be able to:

1. Outline the process for reconstituting commercial powdered formula.
2. Identify potential genetic or neurological factors that could impact infant feeding.
3. Name conditions that may be present that warrant the need for total parental nutrition.
4. Discuss the importance of postnatal growth in infancy.

FORMULA FEEDING

Whether a mother develops a condition that requires her to stop breastfeeding, or it is her choice to formula feed, support and educate the new family on proper formula preparation and feeding techniques.

Commercial Formulas

Commercial formula preparations are supervised by the Food and Drug Administration. All formulas are designed to simulate the nutritional content of breast milk and contain supplemental vitamins, most commonly iron (Table 9.1).

Forms of Commercial Formulas

- Powder combined with water (lowest cost)
- Condensed liquid diluted with an equal amount of water
- Ready-to-pour formulas
- Individually prepackaged and prepared bottles of formula (highest cost)

Docosahexaenoic Acid and Arachidonic Acid

- Docosahexaenoic acid (DHA) and arachidonic acid (ARA) are fatty acids naturally passed from mother to fetus in pregnancy and are naturally occurring in breast milk.
- All infant formulas sold in the United States use the same sources of DHA and ARA.
- DHA and ARA are thought to aid in the development and possibly promote of the infant's brain and eyesight.

Table 9.1

Different Types of Formulas	
Milk-based formulas	For most full-term newborns
Lactose-free formulas	For infants with lactose intolerance or galactosemia
Soy formulas	For infants allergic to cow's milk protein
Elemental formulas	For infants with protein allergies and fat malnutrition

DHA and ARA are fatty acids naturally found in breast milk that may be important in the development of membrane constituents in the central nervous system and promote eye and brain development.

Calculation of Formula's Adequacy

Total fluid ingested in 24 hours must be sufficient to meet needs; 75 to 90 mL (2.5 to 3 ounces) of fluid per pound of body weight per day (150 to 200 mL/kg) are needed. The number of calories required per day is 50 to 55 calories per pound of body weight (100 to 120 kcal/kg). Add 2 or 3 ounces to the infant's age in months.

Parents often change formulas in response to infant colic or fear that there is an allergic reaction to a specific brand of formula. Most colic improves spontaneously between 4 and 6 months of age. True allergies to protein, on the other hand, will persist and will present not as crying but as diarrhea, vomiting, and anemia in the newborn. In the case of a true allergy, the newborn may need to be switched to a prescribed formula.

Preparation for Formula

- Wash the top of the can with warm, soapy water and rinse.
- Pour into clean bottles.
- Apply nipple; do not touch the nipple.
- Place bottle cap over the nipple and refrigerate.

Formula should never be further diluted as this will reduce its nutritional components. Mothers may intentionally water down powdered formula as a money-saving practice while not fully realizing that this negatively impacts the newborn or infant.

Effective Feeding Techniques

- A microwave will heat formula unevenly (hotter in the center of the bottle than on the sides). Shake bottle and test formula on wrist.
- Do not store and reuse formula.
- Obtain a comfortable position.
- Limit infants to 30-minute feedings so that calories expended overall are greater than the intake of calories.

Fast Facts

New parents should remember to keep the baby's head elevated and to avoid excess intake of air. The newborn should be burped after ingestion of every 10 to 15 ounces. Bottles should never be propped for feedings, as this increases the chance of suffocation.

SPECIALIZED FORMULAS FOR PRETERM INFANTS

Premature infants have increased nutritional needs to support their unique needs. Preterm human milk has higher levels of certain nutrients, yet it still remains below the necessary daily allowances. Breast milk remains the ideal feeding choice as it is associated with improved long-term immunity properties, reduced incidence of necrotizing enterocolitis (NEC), protection against sepsis, earlier discharge, fewer infections in the first year of life, and better feeding tolerance.

Fortification of Human Milk

Fortification of human milk is indicated in infants <1,500 grams. It is sometimes administered to infants between 1,800–2,000 g and to infants younger than 34 gestational weeks, especially when these infants are identified to be at risk for NEC and feeding intolerances. Human milk fortifiers and donor milk fortifiers are available. The fortifier added is 2 to 4 kcal/oz up to 100 mL/day.

Premature Formula

When breast milk is either not available or formula feeding has been chosen as a feeding preference, specialized formula may be used. Preterm formulas are typically whey-based and have increased plasma amino acids, high percentage of carbohydrates to combat lactate deficiency, and higher levels of fat mixtures to compensate for premature pancreatic and bile acid production related to extreme prematurity.

These specialized formulas also have higher levels of vitamins, minerals, proteins, and electrolytes to support growth and reduce fluid tolerance. Formula designed for premature infants typically has higher caloric values per mL to meet the additional nutritional needs of these infants. The carbohydrate mixture is typically 40% to 50% lactase and 50% to 60% glucose polymers, which is adjusted since preterm infants have a lactase deficiency. Most premature infant formulas also have 40% to 50% fat mixtures and 50% to 60% to compensate for the reduced pancreatic secretion and the requirements for additional fatty acids.

Fast Facts

Mothers of premature newborns should begin breast pumping immediately following birth and should continue pumping throughout the newborn's hospitalization. A lactation consultation should be provided prior to discharge to assist the new mother with a pumping schedule, proper milk storage, and guidelines for transporting milk to the hospital for feedings while the infant remains in the NICU.

TOTAL PARENTERAL NUTRITION

Total parenteral nutrition (TPN) is commonly used in infants <1,500 g to ensure adequate caloric, amino acid, and nitrogen balance. TPN also reduces the expenditure of excess calories in preterm and low-birth-weight infants. The use of TPN is considered when oral feedings are not likely to be initiated within the next 3 to 5 days or if a cardiac condition is present that would necessitate calcium supplementation. TPN can be administered via a peripheral route, central route, or via the umbilical vein. While central TPN can support more hypertonic solution concentrations, it is associated with higher infection rates. Central line administration may be considered under the following situations (Eichenwald, Hansen, Martin, & Stark, 2017):

- Lack of peripheral or umbilical access
- Duration of treatment likely to exceed 7 days
- Excess nutritional needs that cannot be supported via the peripheral route

FEEDING RECOMMENDATIONS FOR INFANTS WITH SPECIAL NEEDS

Prematurity

Premature infants have increased nutritional needs. The quantity of nutritional source is largely determined by the newborn's weight. As the weight and ability to tolerate oral feedings increases, the volume is increased as tolerated, typically 2 to 4 kcal/oz prior to reaching 100 mL/kg/day. Once the volume is increased, it is typically maintained at that volume for 24 hours. If the new volume is tolerated, advancement is recommended every 24 hours. As premature infant diets are advanced, it is important to closely monitor total daily fluid levels to prevent fluid overload.

Oral Anatomical Issues

Feeding and swallowing may be difficult due to anatomical defects that interfere with the ability to form an adequate seal needed for sucking and swallowing. Defects, pain from surgical interventions, and lack of experience may interfere with the ability to adequately feed. Specialized nipples are available to aid infants with cleft lips and cleft palates in bottle-feeding (Gottschlich et al., 2018).

Neurological Issues

Neurological brain malformations may make feeding difficult. Lack of coordination, presence of abnormal movements, or an inability to suck and swallow can result from a neurological abnormality.

Genetic Issues

Feeding and swallowing difficulties are common in infants with genetic defects and can be a combination of etiological factors including medical, physiological, anatomical, or behavioral. Feeding may be uncomfortable, painful, or difficult as a result of choking, gagging, emesis, regurgitation, or other symptoms that may occur as a result of various genetic issues. Neuromotor impairments may include open mouth posture, hypotonia, and lack of coordinated tongue movements (Briere, McGrath, Cong, Brownell, & Cusson, 2016).

INTERVENTIONS FOR INFANTS WITH SPECIAL NEEDS

Although infants with special needs would benefit greatly from the immune-benefits of human breast milk, the incidence of breastfeeding or the supplementation of expressed breast milk is lower in these high-risk groups. Infants with special needs who have difficulties with feedings require an interdisciplinary approach to manage their care and assist in developing a safe, realistic feeding program that results in optimal growth. Interdisciplinary team members may include the neonatologist, gastroenterologist, lactation consultant, behavioral psychologist, speech pathologist, and nutritionist.

POSTNATAL GROWTH

Alterations in postnatal growth rates commonly occur in premature infants and warrant special consideration due to a reduced nutritional reserve in preterm infants. Factors associated with prematurity and low birth weight include:

- Poor postnatal growth increases the risk of neurodevelopmental impairment and poor cognitive outcomes.
- Premature growth charts are available for birth weight ranges: 1,500 g or less and 1,501 to 2,500 g (52.95 to 88.18 ounces).
- Variations in newborn growth are based on gestational age, gender, weight, genetics, and coexisting morbidities.
- "Catch-up" growth is generally considered to be achieved when the infant reaches between the 5th and 10th percentiles on a standard growth chart.
- Premature infants' catch-up growth presents first in the head circumference, then in weight and length.
- After 2 years of age, a standard growth chart may be used.

References

Briere, C. E., McGrath, J. M., Cong, X., Brownell, E., & Cusson, R. (2016). Direct-breastfeeding in the neonatal intensive care unit and breastfeeding duration for premature infants. *Applied Nursing Research, 32,* 47–51. doi:10.1016/j.apnr.2016.04.004

Eichenwald, E. C., Hansen, A. R., Martin, C. R., & Stark, A. R. (2017). *Cloherty and Stark's manual of neonatal care* (8th ed.). Philadelphia, PA: Wolters Kluwer.

Gottschlich, M. M., Mayes, T., Allinger C., James, L., Khoury, J., Pan, B., & van Aalst, J. A. (2018). A retrospective study identifying breast milk feeding disparities in infants with cleft palate. *Journal of the Academy of Nutrition and Dietetics, 118*(11), 2154–2161. doi:10.1016/j.jand.2018.05.008

IV

Common Neonatal Conditions and Infections

10

Respiratory Alterations

Certain conditions occur commonly in the newborn period. Respiratory alterations are among the most commonly occurring disorders in the immediate neonatal period and warrant prompt identification and intervention.

Nurses working with newborns need to have a comprehensive understanding of the pathophysiological processes that put a newborn at risk for certain commonly occurring respiratory conditions. Prompt identification of adverse conditions and proper nursing care to identify specific complications and prevent further complications are required.

During this part of the orientation, the nurse will be able to:

1. Compare and contrast the differences between newborn asphyxia and hypoxia.
2. Outline appropriate nursing interventions for respiratory distress.
3. Describe the adverse effects associated with apnea related to prematurity.
4. Discuss the potential complications related to meconium aspiration syndrome.
5. Identify potential long-term effects that may occur as a reperfusion injury.

ASPHYXIA

Asphyxia refers to a deprivation of oxygen (hypoxia), which commonly results from a drop in maternal blood pressure or interference with blood flow to the fetal brain during delivery. This can occur from inadequate circulation or perfusion, impaired respiratory effort, or inadequate ventilation after birth.

Possible Etiological Factors

When the placenta does not provide the fetus with enough oxygen, fetal hypoxia will result. Symptoms of low fetal oxygen states include:

- Meconium-stained amniotic fluid and umbilical cord
- Late fetal heart rate decelerations
- Bradycardia
- Prolonged labor
- Breech birth
- Placental abruption
- Maternal sedation in preterm infants

Fast Facts

Even though asphyxia and fetal hypoxia are not the same, fetal hypoxia is the most common cause of asphyxia.

HYPOXIA

Hypoxia, a condition in which the body is deprived of adequate oxygen, commonly occurs when the newborn fails to breathe adequately after delivery.

Potential Etiological Factors

- Prematurity
- Cord prolapse
- Cord occlusion
- Placental infarction
- Intrauterine growth restriction
- Maternal smoking

RESPIRATORY DISTRESS

Transient Tachypnea of the Newborn

Transient tachypnea of the newborn (TTN; "transient" means temporary; "tachypnea" means fast breathing rate) is a term for a mild newborn respiratory problem that begins soon after birth and can last up to 3 days. Only a small percentage of all newborns develop TTN. Most babies with this problem are full term, although premature infants can also develop TTN.

Possible Etiological Factors

- Slow absorption of fluid in the fetal lungs
- Cesarean birth

Adverse Effects

- Tachypnea (over 60 breaths/minute)
- Grunting sounds with breathing
- Flaring of the nostrils
- Retractions

Nursing Considerations

Treatment for transient tachypnea of the newborn depends on gestational age, overall health, and medical history, as well as the extent of the condition and the newborn's tolerance for specific medications, procedures, or therapies. Treatment options may include:

- Chest X-ray for diagnostic purposes
- Supplemental oxygen given by mask or oxygen hood
- Ongoing oxygen monitoring
- Continuous positive airway pressure (CPAP) treatment
- Mechanical ventilation
- Tube feedings

APNEA

Apnea in the newborn period in term infants is described as the cessation of respirations for a period of 20 or more seconds or a period of cessation of breathing associated with bradycardia, cyanosis, pallor, or hypotonia.

In premature infants, the most common type of apnea is the cessation of breathing for 20 seconds with bradycardia or a reduction of oxygen saturation. Central apnea is due to the depression of the respiratory center and is marked by a cessation of output from the respiratory centers. Obstructive apnea occurs with airway obstruction, and respiratory efforts do not maintain ventilation. Mixed apnea, a combination of central and obstructive apnea, is most common in preterm infants.

Adverse Effects

- Hypoxia
- Cyanosis
- Hypercarbia
- Respiratory arrest
- Respiratory failure

Nursing Considerations

Determination of risk at the time of birth is important, especially the identification of prematurity. Assess the need for immediate resuscitation to stabilize the newborn. After an apnea episode, infants should be admitted to the high-risk observation unit or NICU for cardiorespiratory and pulse oximetry monitoring. Infants with apnea of prematurity warrant interventions for frequent or prolonged apnea episodes since they need frequent stimulation. If an apnea episode occurs, flick the foot or rub the back to stimulate spontaneous respirations. Nasal CPAP and methylxanthine therapy may be necessary.

MECONIUM ASPIRATION SYNDROME

Meconium aspiration syndrome occurs when the newborn aspirates meconium into the lungs by breathing in a mixture of meconium and amniotic fluid at the time of birth.

Adverse Effects

- Cyanosis
- Respiratory distress

- Nasal flaring
- Grunting
- Low Apgar scores
- Abnormal breath sounds
- Acidosis
- Infection

Nursing Considerations

Once meconium-stained amniotic fluid is identified, oral suctioning is performed when the head is on the perineum prior to the delivery of the body. For thick meconium, a laryngoscope suctions the airway and prevents aspiration. Respiratory support and possible resuscitation may be required. Ongoing respiratory depression warrants a chest X-Ray to observe for blockages and pneumothorax. The infant is placed in a warmer to maintain body temperature. Most infants do well, but some may require CPAP or warrant support on a ventilator. Surfactant is sometimes administered along with antibiotics. Close monitoring for persistent pulmonary hypertension is warranted.

REPERFUSION INJURY

A second stage of damage called "reperfusion injury" occurs after the restoration of normal blood flow and reoxygenation to the brain due to the release of toxins by damaged cells. The degree of injury varies. Infants with mild or moderate asphyxia may have a full recovery, whereas infants who had prolonged oxygen deprivation may have permanent injury to the brain, heart, lungs, bowels, kidneys, or other organs.

Adverse Effects

Outcomes of newborns affected with asphyxia and hypoxia vary. Premature infants are at greatest risk to experience adverse effects, which may include:

- Heart rate variations
- Respiratory distress
- Central cyanosis
- Hypotonia
- Cerebral palsy
- Developmental disabilities
- Attention deficit hyperactivity disorder
- Impaired sight

- Complete organ failure
- Death

Nursing Considerations

Good management during labor and delivery and the early detection of nonreassuring fetal status are the best methods of preventing asphyxia. However, some cases of asphyxia cannot be predicted or prevented. In that case, asphyxia and the subsequent prevention of prolonged hypoxia require resuscitating the newborn infant. Only about 5% of newborn infants have asphyxia and require resuscitation.

11

Common Neonatal Conditions

The early newborn period marks a dramatic transition from intrauterine to extrauterine life. Early neonatal conditions, such as cold stress and hypoglycemia, can occur in the first few hours after birth. Ongoing assessment is needed to ensure that the newborn is adapting appropriately after birth. Jaundice is common in many newborns, but when it occurs in the first 24 hours can warrant more intensive assessment, laboratory studies, and interventions. Persistent pulmonary hypertension requires intensive care and monitoring.

During this part of the orientation, the nurse will be able to:

1. Identify adverse outcomes that may occur as a result of cold stress.
2. Determine risk factors for hypoglycemia that warrant blood sugar monitoring in the immediate newborn period.
3. Explain the pathophysiological process that leads to newborn jaundice.
4. List the criteria for bilirubin toxicity in the newborn.
5. Describe interventions for the newborn with persistent pulmonary hypertension.

COLD STRESS

Cold stress is the inability to maintain a core body temperature, resulting in a markedly decreased body temperature (hypothermia) and an increased metabolic rate. Cold stress occurs most commonly in low-birth-weight and very-low-birth-weight (VLBW) infants. An estimated 27.8% of VLBW infants experience cold stress (Bissinger & Annibale, 2010).

Glucose is necessary in larger amounts when the metabolic rate rises to produce heat; if the glycogen stores are depleted or were sparse to begin with, hypoglycemia may result. Hypoglycemia in combination with the metabolism of brown fat causes the release of fatty acids, leading to acidosis. From there, the elevated fatty acids can interfere with the transport of bilirubin to the liver, leading to an increased risk of jaundice. When acidosis occurs and the body attempts to conserve heat, vasoconstriction occurs and the risk of pulmonary vasoconstriction opening the patent ductus arteriosus occurs. Reverting back to fetal circulation can lead to hypoxia and can influence the left-to-right shunting, thereby increasing respiratory distress.

Hazards of Cold Stress

- Increased need for oxygen
- Respiratory distress
- Decreased surfactant production
- Hypoglycemia
- Metabolic acidosis
- Jaundice

Possible Etiological Factors

- Prematurity
- Growth-restricted infants
- Infants with asphyxia
- Infants with respiratory difficulties
- Poor environmental conditions (where heat loss is likely to occur)

Signs & Symptoms

- Temperature below 97.5°F (36.4°C)
- Weak cry
- Lethargic
- Reddish, cool skin
- Cool extremities and abdomen

- Feeding difficulties
- Hypoglycemia

Adverse Effects

Ongoing cold stress can lead to:

- Hypoglycemia
- Burning of brown fat
- Impaired weight gain
- Metabolic acidosis
- Newborn jaundice

Nursing Considerations for Infants With Cold Stress

The best method of handling cold stress is prevention. Interventions to reduce cold stress include:

- Preventing drafts and temperature changes in the delivery room area
- Observing for signs of cold stress
- Maintaining a neutral thermal environment (NTE)
- Monitoring and assessing skin temperature every 15 to 20 minutes
- Warming the baby slowly
- Increasing hourly temperature by 33.8°F (1°C) per hour until the temperature stabilizes
- Obtaining blood sugar to determine whether hypoglycemia is present
- Warming IV fluids prior to administration
- Avoiding heat loss through evaporation, convection, conduction, and radiation

Neutral Thermal Environment

An NTE is the environment in which the body temperature is within the recommended range. The NTE allows for minimal oxygen and caloric consumption and the least metabolic energy expenditure. This can vary depending on the infant's age and weight. Nurses can maintain an NTE by:

- Providing external heat sources (radiant warmers, isolettes, k-pads, etc.)
- Avoiding cold exposure during procedures such as bathing and diapering
- Keeping the infant's head covered
- Swaddling the infant to conserve heat
- Keeping the infant in a flexed position to optimize warmth

Glucose levels should be closely monitored after glucose supplementation (orally or IV) to evaluate whether the hypoglycemia
occurs again.

HYPERBILIRUBINEMIA (JAUNDICE)

Jaundice refers to the yellow pigmentation of the skin and conjunctival membranes caused by excess bilirubin in the blood; it occurs
when the old cells break down and hemoglobin is changed into bilirubin and removed by the liver. It is estimated that over 50% of newborns will develop some amount of jaundice during the first week of
life. The buildup of bilirubin in the blood is called *hyperbilirubinemia*. See Table 11.1 for different types of jaundice.

Table 11.1

Types of Jaundice	
Physiologic jaundice	Occurs as a "normal" response to the baby's limited ability to excrete bilirubin in the first days of life; occurs after 24 hours of life; most of the time resolves without treatment.
Pathologic jaundice	Jaundice may occur with the abnormal breakdown of red blood cells due to hemolytic disease of the newborn (Rh disease), polycythemia (too many red blood cells), inadequate liver function, infection, or other factors; occurs within first 24 hours of life; needs additional medical management and may be associated with infection or congenital defect. Neonatal hypoxia and reduced bowel motility are also common causes.
Breast milk jaundice	Jaundice that is common in breastfed infants occurring between 5–14 days of life related to increased concentrations of beta-glucuronidase in breast milk, causing an increase in the deconjugation and reabsorption of bilirubin.
Breastfeeding jaundice	Jaundice occurs in 15% of infants due to low breast milk intake, dehydration, and low calorie intake. The lack of formation of bacteria in the gastrointestinal tract is thought to result in a reduced ability of the body to absorb metabolites into bilirubin for proper secretion.

Possible Etiological Factors

- Prematurity
- Maternal–fetal incompatibility
- Cephalhematoma
- Areas of bruising
- Feeding problems
- Cold stress
- Toxoplasmosis infection during pregnancy
- Gestational diabetes
- Birth trauma
- Delayed cord clamping

Fast Facts

The timing of the appearance of jaundice helps with the diagnosis. Bilirubin level peaks in a term baby at 3 to 5 days and in 5 to 7 days in a preterm baby.

Familial Risk Factors

Certain infants are at an increased risk of developing jaundice based on family history. These risk factors include family members with:

- Previous sibling with jaundice
- Eastern Asian, Greek, and Native American descent
- Anemia
- Gallbladder disease
- Splenomegaly
- G6PD deficiency
- Liver Disease

Fast Facts

Although low levels of bilirubin are not usually a concern, large amounts can circulate to tissues in the brain and may cause seizures and brain damage. This condition is called *kernicterus*.

Signs & Symptoms

- Yellow coloring of the baby's skin, usually beginning on the face and moving down the body

- Yellowing of the sclera
- Poor feeding
- Pallor

Adverse Effects

- Listlessness
- High-pitched cry
- Difficulty arousing
- Feeding difficulties
- Arching backward
- Kernicterus
- Chronic bilirubin encephalopathy

Nursing Considerations for Infants With Jaundice

Treatment depends on many factors, including the cause of the jaundice, the level of bilirubin, the extent of the disease, gestational age, overall health, and medical history. The goal is to keep the level of bilirubin from increasing to dangerous levels. Key nursing interventions include:

- Identification of infants at risk
- Frequent nursing to maintain hydration and aid in excretion
- Maintaining thermoregulation
- Phototherapy
- Fiber optic blanket
- Exchange transfusion
- Increased breastfeeding
- Treatment of underlying conditions

Fast Facts

Maintain the baby's temperature to decrease stress and acidosis, monitor stools for frequency, and encourage early breastfeeding and adequate and frequent hydration via feedings to promote intestinal colonization and calories needed for hepatic binding proteins.

PATHOLOGIC JAUNDICE

Pathologic jaundice warrants intensive treatment as it has the potential to result in bilirubin toxicity; it is not considered a normal neonatal response to extrauterine life.

Indicators of Pathological Jaundice

- Jaundice occurs in the first 24 hours or after 7 days
- Jaundice continues beyond 2 weeks
- Rise in total serum bilirubin >0.2 mg/dL
- Bilirubin level increases of 5 mg/dL per day
- Bilirubin levels >18 mg/dL
- Evidence of infection

Possible Etiological Factors

- Immune hemolytic anemia
- Nonimmune hemolytic anemia
- Sepsis
- Hypothyroidism
- Polycythemia
- Rh disease
- Liver abnormality
- Gastrointestinal obstruction
- Congenital heart disease
- Metabolic disorder
- Bleeding disorder
- Hypothyroidism

HYPERBILIRUBINEMIA TREATMENTS

Phototherapy

Phototherapy is typically the initial intervention for infants with hyperbilirubinemia. Home phototherapy with bilirubin blankets is not as effective as overhead phototherapy lights but may be an acceptable form of treatment for infants that meet preset criteria and have physiological jaundice. It is not an appropriate therapy for pathological jaundice. The nurse ensures the neonate is properly assessed throughout the intervention by providing the following interventions:

- Place in an isolate (or rarely a crib) for thermal environmental stability.
- Place opaque eye patches.
- Ensure eye patches are not occluding nose.
- Remove clothing and blankets with diaper in place.
- Monitor vital signs every 4 hours.
- Strictly monitor intake and output.
- Weigh all diapers.
- Weigh daily.

- Reposition to ensure full light exposure and prevent pressure areas.
- Cluster care activities with parent visits.
- Remove eye patches and assess with feedings every 2 to 3 hours.
- Uninterrupted phototherapy for all feedings until levels fall below 20 mg/dL, then breastfeeding and expressed breastmilk can be given by parents for brief periods of time.
- Supplemental breastmilk or formula should be given if excessive weight loss or dehydration is occurring.
- Discontinue lights during blood draws.
- If initiated during hospitalization after birth, initial blood draw is at 4 to 6 hours after initiation and then every 8 to 12 hours per agency policy if steadily declining. More frequent intervals are warranted if abnormal or slower-than-expected decline in levels.
- Assess placement of bilirubin blanket under infant.
- If initiated due to readmission, monitor at 2 to 3 hours after initiation.
- Montior 18 to 24 hours after discontinuing therapy to ensure elevations and continued reductions in levels are occurring.

Exchange Transfusions

Exchange transfusions are warranted to reduce abnormally high bilirubin levels or when phototherapy fails and toxic levels are present. Exchange transfusions are also indicted for newborns with Rh disease. The goal of exchange transfusions is to decrease the bilirubin levels by 50%. A rebound of up to 60% posttransfusion is common. With exchange transfusions, fresh O negative irradiated packed red blood cells (PRBC) are usually transfused via an umbilical venous catheter, with either one double-volume transfusion of 160 mL/kg transfused over 2 to 4 hours or two transfusions of 80 mL/kg over 1 to 2 hours is performed. The blood is administered via a blood warmer to maintain a temperature of 37°C. Albumin is infused prior to the transfusion to facilitate the removal of bilirubin. The infant is placed back in phototherapy after the transfusion with serum monitoring at 2, 4, and 6 hours and at least every 12 to 24 hours thereafter. Repeat transfusions are sometimes indicted based on bilirubin levels.

BILIRUBIN TOXICITY

Bilirubin toxicity occurs when bilirubin is deposited into the brain and results in bilirubin-induced neurologic dysfunction (BIND).

It is more common when bilirubin levels exceed 25 mg/dL and in late preterm and term infants. The stages of BIND are presented in Table 11.2.

Kernicterus

Kernicterus is an adverse outcome of BIND and is a permanent condition that develops during the first year of life following bilirubin toxicity.

Symptoms of Kernicterus

- Hearing loss
- Dental enamel dysphagia
- Limited upward gaze
- Neuromotor impairment
- Choreoathetoid cerebral palsy

Table 11.2

Phases of BIND	
Early Phase	Lethargy
	High-pitched cry
	Poor feeding
	Poor sucking reflex
	Hypotonia
Intermediate Phase	Hypertonia
	Oculogyric crisis
	Fever
	Irritability
	Kernicterus
	Death
Advanced Phase	Opisthotonus
	Retrocollis
	Shrill or weak cry
	Apnea
	Seizures
	Respiratory failure
	Death

RESPIRATORY DISTRESS

Transient Tachypnea of the Newborn

Transient tachypnea of the newborn (TTN; "transient" means temporary; "tachypnea" means fast breathing rate) is a term for a mild newborn respiratory problem that begins soon after birth and can last up to 3 days. Only a small percentage of all newborns develop TTN. Most babies with this problem are full term, although premature infants can also develop TTN.

Possible Etiological Factors

- Slow absorption of fluid in the fetal lungs
- Cesarean birth

Signs & Symptoms

- Tachypnea (over 60 breaths/minute)
- Grunting sounds with breathing
- Flaring of the nostrils
- Retractions

Adverse Effects

- Increased respiratory effort
- Respiratory distress
- Cyanosis

Nursing Considerations for Infants With TTN

Treatment for TTN depends on gestational age, overall health, and medical history, as well as the extent of the condition and the newborn's tolerance for specific medications, procedures, or therapies. Treatment options may include:

- Chest X-ray for diagnostic purposes
- Supplemental oxygen given by mask or oxygen hood
- CPAP treatment
- Mechanical ventilation
- Tube feedings
- Laboratory assessments (CBC, cultures)
- Chest X-Ray (if symptoms do not subside)

PERSISTENT PULMONARY HYPERTENSION

Persistent pulmonary hypertension (PPHN) is also known as persistent fetal circulation. The incidence of PPHN is approximately 1 to 2 in every 1,000 live births. In this condition, a newborn circulatory system reverts back to fetal circulation due to lowered oxygen levels or difficulty breathing at birth (Hansen, Eichenwald, Stakr, & Martin, 2016).

Possible Etiological Factors

- Full-term or post-term pregnancies
- Pulmonary parenchymal diseases
- Congenital respiratory tract malformations
- Cardiac abnormalities
- Pneumonia, sepsis
- Traumatic birth
- Birth asphyxia

Signs & Symptoms

- Grunting
- Nasal flaring
- Tachypnea
- Increased anterior-posterior chest circumference
- Cyanosis
- Gradient of >10% in oxygen saturation between preductal and postductal arterial blood gases (ABGs)

Adverse Effects

- Cyanosis
- Tachypnea
- Tachycardia
- Low blood oxygen levels, even while receiving 100% oxygen

Nursing Considerations for Infants With PPHN

Treatment of PPHN is aimed at increasing oxygen to the rest of the body systems; however, long-term health problems may be related to damage from lowered oxygen in the body. Assessments are performed by obtaining an electrocardiogram with doppler studies. The chest X-ray will be either normal or show RV predominance.

Treatment for PPHN may include:

- 100% supplemental oxygen by mask or hood
- Endotracheal tube and mechanical ventilation
- Nitric oxide (to help dilate the blood vessels in the lungs)
- Pharmacological interventions may include volume expanders, sedatives, analgesics, vasopressors, hydrocortisone, and afterload reducers.

- Administration of iNO via inhalation at initial doses of 20 ppm to decrease PVR with gradual taper as respiratory improvement occurs
- Extracorporeal membrane oxygenation (ECMO)—cardiopulmonary bypass during which oxygen is added and carbon dioxide is removed. ECMO is only used in specialized neonatal intensive care units (NICUs).
- Interventions to correct metabolic abnormalities (hypoglycemia and hypocalcemia)
- Partial exchange transfusions if polycythemia is present
- Minimal stimulation during assessments and care
- Continuous vital sign monitoring

References

Bissinger, R. L., & Annibale, D. J. (2010). Thermoregulation in very low birth weight infants during the golden hour. *Advances in Neonatal Care, 10*(5), 230–238. doi:10.1097/ANC.0b013e3181f0ae63

Hansen, A. R., Eichenwald, E. C., Stark, A. C., & Martin, C. R. (2016). *Cloherty & Stark's manual of neonatal care.* St. Louis, MO: Lippincott, Williams, & Wilkins.

12

Common Neonatal Infections

There are a number of infections that can occur in the newborn period. Infections are especially dangerous in the newborn period as the newborn has limited immunological defenses in place. Infections can occur from vertical transmission in the course of pregnancy or during labor and delivery. They can also be contracted in the early newborn period.

During this part of the orientation, the nurse will be able to:

1. Identify potential sources of infection that may be diagnosed in the newborn period.
2. Detail common viral infections that may develop in the newborn period.
3. Discuss potential adverse outcomes associated with group B streptococcus.
4. Describe possible symptoms that may occur in the newborn with sepsis.
5. Outline the treatment for infants with a fungal infection.

Newborn infants have limited ability to prevent and fight infectious diseases. Special care is needed for babies who develop an infection before, during, or after birth. Several infectious sources are briefly reviewed, followed by sections on the most commonly occurring infections. Table 12.1 summarizes other infections that can occur during the perinatal period.

VIRAL INFECTIONS

Viral infections can impact the fetus/neonate when infection occurs through vertical transmission (in utero), during the intrapartum period, or through postnatal infection in the postpartum period. When a viral infection is suspected, diagnostic testing is indicated. A comprehensive review of potential etiologies should be identified so testing can be performed.

Cytomegalovirus (CMV) is the most commonly occurring viral infection and the leading cause of perinatal infection and subsequent disability.

Herpes simplex virus, once responsible for neonatal deaths and disability, has been significantly reduced by aggressive pharmacological treatment.

Pediatric HIV infection can be significantly reduced through the use of perinatal or neonatal antiviral therapy. In developing countries that lack access to these agents, the incidence of infection remains high. Noncompliance with antiviral therapy in pregnancy and in the postpartum period can result in increased pediatric HIV rates.

Hepatitis B can be largely reduced by proper immunizations and immunoglobin treatment.

Respiratory Syncytial Virus

Respiratory syncytial virus (RSV) is a viral illness that often mimics a cold and is the most common cause of bronchiolitis and pneumonia. It is frequently found in NICUs. Although the virus does not typically occur until 1 month of age, premature babies are at an increased risk for infection. The incubation period is 4 days (Eichenwald, Hansen, Martin, & Stark, 2017). RSV is more common in the winter and spring months in the United States.

Possible Etiological Factors

- Spread from respiratory secretions of the eyes, mouth, or nose
- Spread through the inhalation of droplets via sneezing or coughing
- Spread through contact with contaminated objects or surfaces
- Infants with chronic lung disease are at greater risk

Signs & Symptoms

- Nasal discharge
- Apnea
- Listlessness
- Fever

- Poor feeding
- Wheezing
- Retractions
- Tachycardia
- Dry, hacking cough

Adverse Effects

- Severe respiratory illness
- Pneumonia, which can become life-threatening
- Development of reactive airway disease (in later life)
- Childhood asthma

Nursing Considerations for Infants With RSV

A review of family history is important because diagnosis is aided by a history of illness in other family members, other babies in the hospital nursery, or the time of year. A swab of the baby's respiratory secretions may show the presence of a virus. Although there are no medications used to treat the virus itself, care of a baby with RSV involves treating the symptoms. Because RSV is caused by a virus, antibiotics are not useful. Interventions may include:

- Supplemental oxygen
- IV fluids
- Tube feedings
- Bronchodilator medications
- Antiviral medications (for very sick or high-risk babies)

One of the following medications (these are not vaccines and do not prevent the virus) is usually given monthly during the RSV season (late fall through spring) to high-risk newborns to lessen the severity of the illness and help shorten the hospital stay:

- Palivizumab, an antibody against RSV
- Respiratory syncytial virus immune globulin IV (RSV-IGIV)

HIV

Perinatal transmission of HIV occurs when the fetus/newborn becomes affected with the HIV virus during pregnancy, labor, or birth, or via breastfeeding.

National Institutes of Health HIV Statistics

- In 2018, 5,000 HIV-positive women gave birth.
- Women with HIV who take antiretroviral medication during pregnancy can reduce transmission rates to less than 1%.

- Transmission risks are approximately 25% in untreated HIV-positive women.
- Transmission rates of 10% to 20% occur during labor and delivery when antiretrovirals are not administered.
- Transmission rates associated with breastfeeding are 15% at 24 months of age.
- Although the number of women with HIV giving birth is increasing, perinatal transmission rates are decreasing (National Institutes of Health [NIH], 2012).
- Perinatal transmission has decreased by 90% since the 1990s as a result of universal screening recommendations and antiretroviral medication (NIH, 2012).

Possible Etiological Factors

- Lack of antiretroviral drug administration in pregnancy, labor, or delivery
- Premature rupture of membranes
- Invasive birth procedures
- Vaginal birth in women with high viral loads
- Instrument/operative vaginal birth

Signs & Symptoms

- Failure to thrive
- Abdominal distention
- Weight loss
- Swollen lymph nodes
- Diarrhea
- Thrush
- Fevers

Adverse Effects

- Enlarged liver and spleen
- Pneumonia
- Infection
- Failure to gain weight
- Hepatitis
- Bacterial infections
- Kidney disease

Nursing Considerations for Infants With HIV

- Offer HIV testing for all infants with undocumented maternal HIV status.
- Obtain referral to social services referral.
- Obtain baseline complete blood count (CBC).

- Begin neonatal zidovudine (ZDV) therapy for the first 6 weeks in newborns whose mothers received antivirals during pregnancy.
- If pharmacological intervention was initiated only during labor and not during pregnancy, the following treatment is recommended:
  - Administer neonatal dose of nevirapine at time of birth, within 48 hours of birth, and 96 hours after second dose.
  - Administer ZDV immediately at the time of birth and continue for 6 weeks.

- Once infants begin pharmacological intervention, hemoglobin and neutrophil counts should be performed 4 to 6 weeks after therapy.
- If HIV status is not established until after birth, administer ZDV for 6 weeks.
- HIV-1 DNA polymerase chain reaction assay should be performed at 14 to 21 days after birth, at 1 to 2 months, and again at 4 to 6 months of age.
- HIV-1 virologic assay is the definitive test for confirmation of HIV status.
- Most infants can be diagnosed by 3 months of age.
- If HIV-1 virologic assay result is positive, immediate referral to an HIV specialist is warranted.
- *Pneumocystis* pneumonia prophylaxis is initiated after the ZDV course is completed and should continue until 12 months of age.
- Assess maternal tuberculosis (TB) status and initiate screening for congenital TB.
- Compassionate parental education and support should be provided.
- Refer to a pediatric provider familiar with caring for infants of HIV-positive mothers.
- Educate to prevent opportunistic infection.
- Encourage HIV testing for family members.
- Breastfeeding is contraindicated in HIV-positive women (in the United States and developed countries).

Fast Facts

The most up-to-date website for HIV/AIDS management should be consulted for HIV treatment recommendations, which can be accessed at http://aidsinfo.nih.gov.

BACTERIAL INFECTIONS

Bacterial infections carry the greatest risk for early-onset sepsis in both term and preterm infants. Group B streptococcus is the most common source for sepsis in the neonatal population. Symptoms of bacterial infection often occur in the intrapartum fever resulting in maternal fever and fetal tachycardia. Prematurity, prolonged rupture of membranes (>18 hours), and low birth weight are also risk factors. Chorioamnionitis is a common finding and warrants prompt treatment with antibiotic therapy. Other causative agents include *Escherichia coli*, viridans streptococci, *Enterococcus*, *Klebsiella*, *Listeria*, *Pseudomonas*, *Staphylococcus aureus*, and *Haemophilus spp.*

Group B Streptococcus

Group B streptococcus (GBS) is a bacteria normally found in the digestive tract, urinary tract, and genital area of both males and females. In fact, one out of every four or five pregnant women carries GBS in her rectum or vagina. Newborns can contract GBS both during pregnancy and from the mother's genital tract during labor and delivery.

Adverse Effects

- Respiratory problems
- Changes in blood pressure
- Neurological problems, such as seizures
- Pneumonia
- Meningitis

Nursing Considerations for Infants With GBS

Possible treatment interventions for infants infected with GBS typically include:

- IV antibiotics; other treatments and specialized care
- NICU care

Fast Facts

About 1 in every 100 to 200 babies whose mothers carry GBS develop symptoms of GBS disease. Nearly 75% of GBS cases among newborns occur in the first week of life, which is called early-onset disease. Premature babies are more susceptible to GBS infection than full-term babies.

Sepsis

Sepsis, also called sepsis neonatorum or neonatal septicemia, is a bacterial infection of the newborn. It develops from microorganisms such as bacteria, viruses, fungi, and parasites. Centers for Disease Control and Prevention statistics show that sepsis affects up to 4 in every 1,000 live births. Newborns acquire infection in one of two ways: vertical transmission (in utero) or horizontal transmission (after birth).

Possible Etiological Factors

- Premature rupture of the membranes
- Prolonged rupture of membranes (greater than 24 hours)
- Bleeding problems
- Traumatic birth
- Chorioamnionitis
- Infection of the placental tissues
- Maternal fever

Babies in the NICU are at increased risk for acquiring nosocomial (hospital-acquired) infections. Most babies in the NICU are high risk and have immature or inadequate immune systems. This makes them more susceptible to infection and more likely to need invasive treatments and procedures. Microorganisms that normally live on the skin may cause infection if they enter the body through catheters and other tubes inserted into the infant's body (Table 12.1). Prematurity, colonization with *Group beta streptococcus* (GBS), intrapartum fever, chorioamnionitis, and prolonged rupture of membranes are all risk factors for neonatal sepsis. Late-onset sepsis occurs 8 to 90 days after birth and is frequently the result of community-acquired infections in term infants or nosocomial infections in preterm infants in the NICU setting. The most common organisms associated with late-onset sepsis are GBS and *Klebsiella* spp.

Adverse Effects

- Temperature instability (usually presents with low temperatures, rather than high)
- Respiratory problems
- Feeding intolerance
- Lethargy
- Hypoglycemia
- Apnea or difficulty breathing
- Bradycardia
- Jaundice

Table 12.1

Common Microorganisms		
Prenatal	**During Delivery**	**After Birth**
Rubella (German measles)	Group B streptococcus (GBS)	Respiratory syncytial virus (RSV)
Cytomegalovirus (CMV)	E. coli	Candida
Varicella zoster virus	Herpes simplex virus Chlamydia trachomatis	Haemophilus influenzae type B (Hib)
Listeria monocytogenes		Enteroviruses
Congenital syphilis		Oral Candida infection
Gonorrhea		Varicella zoster virus
Herpes		Enteroviruses
Congenital Zika syndrome		GBSC
Chlamydia trachomatis		Klebsiella spp
Parvovirus B19		
Hepatitis B & C		
NANB viral hepatitis (HEV)		
Hepatitis G (HGV)		
Varicella zoster virus		
Enteroviruses		
Toxoplasmosis		
Syphilis		

Nursing Considerations for Infants With Sepsis

A sepsis workup may be needed to help identify the location of the infection and type of microorganism causing the infection. A sepsis workup and treatment may include the following:

- Laboratory testing—blood cultures, urine samples, complete blood count, cerebrospinal fluid, C-reactive protein
- Application of broad-spectrum antibiotics
- Application of ampicillin and gentamicin
- Supportive care

  - IV fluids
  - Oxygen
  - Temperature stabilization
  - Glucose stabilization

FUNGAL INFECTIONS

Fungal infections rarely cause serious diseases and are nearly always related to *Candida* infections. Contamination within the birth canal, through touch (hands) by the mother, or via breastfeeding may occur prior to the colonization of normal intestinal flora in the newborn's intestinal tract, which can lead to infection in the newborn. The most common infection is oral candidiasis, which is treated with oral nystatin solution. Fluconazole may be used if nystatin is ineffective or in an immunocompromised infant.

Systemic candidiasis is rare but may occur in very preterm, very-low-birth-weight infants, resulting in candidiasis sepsis, which has a 33% fatality rate.

Invasive Infection Risk Factors

- Birth weight <1,000 g
- Central catheter placement
- Delayed oral feedings
- Broad-spectrum antibiotic use
- Presence of candidiasis dermatitis diaper rash
- Vaginal birth
- Prematurity
- Presence of hypoglycemia and thrombocytopenia
- Use of beta-blockers or systemic steroids

References

Eichenwald, E. C., Hansen, A. R., Martin, C. R., & Stark, A. R. (2017). *Cloherty and Stark's manual of neonatal care* (8th ed.). Philadelphia, PA: Wolters Kluwer.

National Institutes of Health. (2018). *HIV and child birth*. Bethesda, MD: National Institutes of Health.

V

High-Risk Neonatal Conditions

13

Adverse Conditions in Very Preterm Neonates (Less Than 32 Weeks)

Preterm birth occurring prior to 32 gestational weeks may put the infant at risk for both short-term and long-term outcomes. The need for ongoing assessment and comprehensive care management is essential for this vulnerable population. Nurses working with premature newborns need to provide extensive clinical care along with education and support.

During this part of the orientation, the nurse will be able to:

1. List the different key terms for prematurity related to gestational age.
2. Discuss possible adverse outcomes associated with premature birth.

PREMATURITY

Occurring in 12% of births in the United States, *prematurity* is defined as a birth that occurs prior to 37 weeks (Davidson, London, & Ladewig, 2020). *Late preterm births* are those that occur between 34 and 36 weeks. Late preterm infants typically have fewer significant long-term complications, they might appear "normal" but are at risk for more adverse outcomes than term infants. *Early preterm birth* refers to births that occur prior to 34 weeks. *Very preterm birth* refers to births that occur prior to 32 weeks. *Extremely preterm birth* refers to births that occur prior to 28 weeks. Extremely preterm neonates often require extensive nursing services and are typically cared for in neonatal intensive care units (NICUs).

Prematurity accounts for 75% to 80% of all neonatal morbidity and mortality (Davidson et al., 2020). Preterm birth is disproportionally increased in Native American and African American populations. Many immediate adverse events associated with prematurity occur in the immediate neonatal period and most commonly occur in infants born prior to 32 gestational weeks. Long-term adverse outcomes are also more common in infants born prior to 32 gestational weeks.

Possible Etiological/Risk Factors

- Congenital birth defects
- Preterm labor
- Low socioeconomic status
- African American race
- Maternal age less than 15 or greater than 40 years of age
- Chorioamnionitis
- Intrauterine growth restriction
- Maternal diabetes
- Multiple gestation
- Tobacco use

Adverse Effects

- Feeding difficulties
- Temperature intolerance
- Infections
- Prolonged jaundice
- Long-term disabilities
- Cerebral palsy
- Neurodevelopmental disabilities
- Pneumonia
- Hearing loss
- Vision deficits
- Intellectual disabilities
- Respiratory distress syndrome
- Bronchopulmonary dysplasia
- Periventricular hemorrhage/intraventricular hemorrhage
- Poorer health and social/emotional functioning measured at preschool age, in adolescence, and in young adulthood

Nursing Considerations for Premature Neonates

- Neonatal resuscitation team should be in attendance for delivery.
- Ensure respiratory stability immediately after birth via respiratory assessment, including pulse oximetry.
- Newborns with respiratory distress may need continuous positive airway pressure (CPAP) given nasally, by mask (Neopuff), or by using an endotracheal tube.
- Surfactant may be administered to accelerate lung maturation (recommend administration within 2 hours of birth).
- Prevent hyperoxia and hypoxia by maintaining oxygen saturation (SaO_2) between 86% and 93%.
- Perform a gestational age assessment at time of birth.
- Ensure temperature stabilization using radiant warmers, incubators, or plastic wrap with a humidified environment for ELBW newborns.
- Monitor blood sugar as needed.
- Skin care should focus on prevention of injury and preventing skin breakdown.
- Maintain adequate intravenous infusions to maintain normal fluid and electrolyte balance.
- Ensure adequate urine output for 24 hours prior to starting electrolyte replacement.
- Assess for jaundice during hospitalization and in the first few days following discharge.
- Monitor weight every 24 hours.
- Educate parents that premature infants may be behind in meeting normal developmental milestones.
- Arrange consultation with developmental pediatrician after discharge.
- Referral to early-intervention services may be warranted in infancy.
- Provide parents with accurate information and support.
- Obtain referrals for support groups or peer mentoring.
- Encourage frequent visitation, phone calls, and sibling visits after mother's discharge to facilitate attachment.
- Assist mother with breast pumping and storage of breast milk during newborn hospitalization.
- Administer car seat safety test prior to discharge.

Fast Facts

The most significant risk factor for preterm birth is a past preterm delivery.

Reference

Davidson, M. R., Ladewig, P. L., & London, M. L. (2020). *Old's maternal-newborn nursing and women's healthcare across the lifespan* (11th ed.). Boston, MA: Pearson Education.

14

Long-Term Sequala of Prematurity

Prematurity can impact the newborn, putting the infant at risk for both short-term and long-term outcomes. The need for ongoing assessment and comprehensive care management is essential for this vulnerable population. Nurses working with premature newborns need to provide extensive clinical care to the newborn along with education and support to the parents.

During this part of the orientation, the nurse will be able to:

1. List the different key terms for prematurity related to gestational age.
2. Discuss possible adverse outcomes associated with prematurity.
3. Analyze the ongoing medical needs of preterm newborns .

PREMATURITY

Occurring in 12% of births in the United States, *prematurity* is defined as a birth that occurs prior to 37 weeks (Davidson, London, & Ladewig, 2020). *Late preterm births* are those that occur between 34 and 36 weeks. Late preterm infants typically have fewer significant long-term complications; they might appear "normal" but are at risk for more adverse outcomes than term infants. *Early preterm births* are those that occur prior to 34 weeks. *Very preterm births* are those that occur prior to 32 weeks. *Extremely preterm births* are those that occur prior to 28 weeks. Extremely preterm neonates often require extensive nursing services and are typically cared for in neonatal intensive care units (NICUs).

Prematurity accounts for 75% to 80% of all neonatal morbidity and mortality (Davidson et al., 2020). Preterm birth is disproportionally increased in the Native American and African American populations. Many immediate adverse events associated with prematurity occur in the immediate neonatal period and most commonly occur in infants born prior to 32 gestational weeks. Long-term adverse outcomes are also more common in infants born prior to 32 gestational weeks.

BRONCHOPULMONARY DYSPLASIA

Bronchopulmonary dysplasia (BPD) is a chronic lung disease, which warrants supplemental oxygen as a result of reduced gas exchange. Infants with persistent oxygen saturation levels below 90% routinely require oxygen.

Symptoms

- Rapid or labored breathing
- Wheezing
- Cyanosis
- Poor growth and development
- Frequent lung infections

Nursing Considerations

- Perform a BPD risk assessment and subsequent hydrocortisone therapy if at ≥60% risk.
- Pharmacology support involves supplementing with:

  - Vitamin A
  - Caffeine citrate
  - Diuretics (if pulmonary retention occurs)
  - Bronchodilators (used to treat bronchospasms, obstructive or chronic increased airway resistance)
  - Pain medications, if needed (sucrose water, morphine, or benzodiazepines)

- Possible mechanical ventilation or oxygen supplementation
- Surfactant replacement therapy
- Fluid management with NaCl and KCl supplements to prevent electrolyte imbalance
- Elevated metabolic rate should be corrected with administration of lipids, which reduces the metabolic rate.

Long-Term Sequela

- Hypertrophic cardiomyopathy
- Intestinal perforation
- Gastric ulcerations can occur with early glucocorticoid therapy
- Pulmonary hypertension
- Systemic hypertension
- Metabolic disturbances from medications
- Systemic to pulmonary shunting
- Infection
- Hearing loss
- Retinopathy of prematurity
- Nephrocalcinosis
- Osteopenia
- Gastrointestinal reflux
- Inguinal hernia
- Failure to thrive

INTRACRANIAL HEMORRHAGE

Hemorrhage occurs into the epidural, subdural, or subarachnoid spaces external to the brain, the parenchyma of the cerebellum or cerebrum, or into the ventricles from the subependymal germinal matrix or choroid plexus.

Symptoms

- Seizures
- Irritability
- Decreased level of consciousness

Nursing Considerations

- Assess for neurological symptoms.
- Ultrasound is commonly used for diagnosis if unstable, otherwise MRI may be obtained.
- Treatment focuses on treating symptoms (pressor support, volume replacement, blood transfusions, anti-convulsant therapy for seizures, surgical intervention is rare).
- Monitor for hydrocephalus, infection, and sinus venous thrombosis.
- Shunt placement may be indicated if post-hemorrhagic ventricular infarction persists for >1 month.

Fast Facts

Ultrasound is indicated for infants <30 gestational weeks between 1 to 2 weeks after birth and again at what would have been 36 to 40 gestational weeks.

Long-Term Sequela

- Hydrocephalus
- Epilepsy
- Hemiparesis
- Cerebral palsy
- Feeding difficulties
- Cognitive impairment
- Ataxia
- Spastic hemiparesis
- Quadriplegia
- Hypotonia
- Tremor
- Nystagmus
- Motor disability
- Death

WHITE MATTER INJURY (PERIVENTRICULAR LEUKOMALACIA)

Diffuse lesions of the white matter extending beyond the periventricular region occurs in <1% of all preterm births.

Symptoms

- Necrosis, gliosis, and disruption in the axons by a hypoxic-ischemic injury, often in the presence of an infectious process

Nursing Considerations

- This is identified in a NICU setting via ultrasound or MRI with an absence of symptoms until several months of age.
- Prevent further white matter injury via stabilization of blood pressure, hemodynamic monitoring, maintaining adequate intravascular volume, oxygenation, and ventilation, and avoiding changes in hemodynamics. Monitor and promptly treat infection.
- Monitor throughout the first year of life; should focus on assessing for spasticity, cognitive, motor or sensory alterations. Targeted therapies are recommended as part of early intervention.

Long-Term Sequela

- Neurodevelopmental defects
- Cerebral palsy
- Diplegia or quadriplegia
- Learning disabilities
- Neurological disabilities
- Neurological impairment
- Vision disturbances
- Vision perception defects

HYPOXIC-ISCHEMIC ENCEPHALOPATHY

Clinical evidence of abnormal neurobehavioral state consists of an altered level of consciousness and symptoms of brainstem or motor dysfunction that are caused by an ischemic-hypoxic injury.

Symptoms

- Altered level of consciousness
- Abnormal infant state (jitteriness, lack of response to stimuli)
- Absence of abnormal newborn reflexes
- Abnormal eye movements: inability to track or failure to blink to bright light

Nursing Considerations

- Assess for symptoms.
- Diagnosis should include a perinatal risk assessment that includes the Apgar scores, umbilical cord blood gases, need for resuscitation at the time of birth, abnormal EEG, or the presence of seizure within 24 hours of birth.

Long-Term Sequela

- Organ dysfunction may occur, which could include acute tubular necrosis.
- Cardiac abnormalities include:

  - ST depression and T-wave inversion, which may indicate reduced left ventricular contractility
  - Right ventricular dysfunction
  - Tricuspid insufficiency
  - Pulmonary hypertension
  - Brain stem injury

- Pulmonary edema
- Pulmonary hemorrhage
- Disseminated intravascular coagulation (DIC)
- Abnormal clotting
- Bone marrow suppression
- Inadequate glycogen storage
- Hyperglycemia
- Slowed metabolism of toxins
- Prolonged excretion of medications
- Risk bowel ischemia
- NEC

SEIZURES

Reduced connectivity in the premature brain and imbalance of excitatory and inhibitory responses due to an excess of overly-inhibited glutamatergic synapses can lead to seizures. Immature systemic processes are associated with altered drug excretion. An abnormal discharge of cortical neurons may result in an epileptic seizure.

Symptoms

- Eyelid fluttering
- Eyes rolling back
- Eyes opening and closing
- Gazing or staring
- Oral smacking
- Sucking or chewing movements
- Protrusion of the tongue
- Abnormal leg movements
- Bicycling leg movements
- Clonic movements
- Abnormal breathing
- Apnea

Nursing Considerations

- Monitor for different types of seizures: subtle, tonic, or clonic.
- Subclinical seizures are only detected by EEG.
- Assess respiratory status as ventilation and oxygenation can become compromised.
- Early diagnosis and identification of the type of seizure should be documented: focal clonic seizures, focal tonic seizures, myoclonic seizures, or autonomic seizures by EEG or bedside EEG.

- Identify underlying etiology, and manage appropriately.
- Treat metabolic needs.
- Supportive respiratory and cardiovascular support is required. Anticonvulsant therapies have risks to premature infants but are often indicated.

Long-Term Sequela

- Benign seizures may carry no long-term risks.
- Long-term outcomes are dependent on the underlying etiology. Gestational age is also a determining factor in long-term adverse events, cerebral palsy, and intellectual disability.

NECROTIZING ENTEROCOLITIS

Acute inflammation injury to the small and large intestines results in necrosis and focal hemorrhage.

Symptoms

- Respiratory distress
- Apnea
- Unstable temperature
- Bloody stools
- Oliguria
- Irritability
- Poor feeding
- Abdominal distention
- Vomiting
- Ileus
- Ascites
- Abdominal mass
- Sepsis

Nursing Considerations

- Assess for risk factors

    - Prematurity
    - Chorioamnionitis
    - IUGR
    - Polycythemia
    - Maternal smoking

- Obtain radiographic studies, which commonly reveal an ileus, mass, and pneumatosis intestinalis.

- Ultrasound with doppler is also indicated.
- Monitor blood cultures, CBC, electrolytes, serial C-reactive protein levels, and stool samples.
- Infants are kept NPO, and IVF are maintained; gastric decompression, and IV antibiotics are administered. With advanced stages, parental nutrition will be indicated along with nasogastric drainage; advanced stages may warrant surgical intervention.

Long-Term Sequela

- Intestinal strictures
- Malabsorption
- Chronic diarrhea
- Dumping syndrome
- Short bowel syndrome
- Fluid and electrolyte loss
- Fistulas
- Hepatitis
- Cholestasis
- Failure to thrive
- Bone disease
- Central nervous system abnormalities
- Cognitive delays or abnormalities

RETINOPATHY OF PREMATURITY (ROP)

Retinopathy is caused by vasoproliferative retinal damage with an increased incidence in lower gestational age and lower birth weight. Prolonged or labile oxygen exposure increases risk of development.

Symptoms

- Myopia
- Nystagmus
- Leukocoria
- Strabismus

Nursing Considerations

- Serial retinal examinations are indicated in infants <30 weeks and for those weighing <1,500 g at birth. The International Classification of Retinopathy of Prematurity is used to classify ROP and to determine appropriate treatment or if ongoing observation and reassessment is indicated.

- Potential treatments

  - Laser therapy
  - Cryotherapy
  - Anti-VEGF therapy
  - Retinal reattachment surgery

Long-Term Sequela

- Altered vision acuity
- Myopia
- Anisometropia
- Astigmatism
- Strabismus
- Amblyopia
- Late retinal detachment
- Glaucoma
- Cicatricial disease

HEARING LOSS

Hearing loss is more common in premature infants and results in delays in language communication and cognitive functioning.

Symptoms

- Lack of startle reflex to sound
- Turning of the head in response to visual but not auditory cues
- Not turning toward sound by 6 months of age
- Lack of any speech by 1 year of age
- Hearing some sounds but not others

Nursing Considerations

- Hearing screening should be conducted prior to 1 month of age via the auditory brainstem response (ABR) method. Abnormal screens require repeat testing. Infants with risk factors for progressive hearing loss or late-onset hearing loss require ongoing monitoring.
- Some infants will require genetic testing.
- Referral to an ophthalmologist is indicated since conditions can co-occur. Referrals to early intervention services, speech therapy, language pathologists, audiologists, and later, special education services are appropriate. Referral to determine if personal amplification systems (hearing aids) are indicated.

If mild hearing loss is detected, referral to an audiologist is warranted. MRI, CT, and radiographic imaging may be ordered.

Long-Term Sequela

- Delayed speech
- Delayed communication
- Cognitive impairment
- Eye abnormalities
- Comorbidities can include

  - Eye disorders
  - Neurological disorders
  - Cariology abnormalities
  - Nephrology issues

OSTEOPENIA

Osteopenia is inadequate postnatal bone mineralization caused by inadequate dietary mineralization, usually low calcium and phosphorus, that results in reduced bone mineralization.

Symptoms

- Inability to wean from ventilator
- Hypotonia
- Painful responses when moving (from underlying fractures)
- Normal head growth with lagging linear growth
- Widened cranial sutures
- Bulging anterior fontanel
- Harrison groves on ribs
- Rachitic rosary
- Enlarged wrists, ankles, and knees

Nursing Considerations

- Assess for risk factors.

  - Birth weight of <800 g
  - Birth prior to 26 weeks
  - Rapidly rising alkaline phosphate

- Perform physical exam.
- Obtain serum phosphorus levels (<3.5 to 4 mg/dL), phosphate activity (>800 IU/L). A combination of phosphorus levels at >4 mg/dL and alkaline phosphate levels at >800 IU/L are suggestive and require diagnostic X-rays to confirm diagnosis. Alkaline phosphate levels at >1,000 IU indicate severe rickets.
- Obtain x-rays of knees and wrists, which show a widening epiphyseal growth plate, fraying, rarefaction of metaphyses, and osteopenia. Treatment aims to establishing oral feedings as soon as feasible with mineral-fortified milk or prepackaged fortifiers; in rare circumstances when supplementing, use both calcium and phosphorus; supplement with vitamin D after infant reaches a weight of 1,500 g and is tolerating oral feedings; monitor calcium, alkaline phosphate and phosphorus levels; use of transitional formula for infants of very low birth weights is recommended; breastfed infants should receive vitamin D supplementation.

Long-Term Sequela

- Fractures
- Long-term osteopenia
- Rickets
- Bone disease

Reference

Davidson, M. R., Ladewig, P. L., & London, M. L. (2020). *Old's maternal-newborn nursing and women's healthcare across the lifespan* (11th ed.). Boston, MA: Pearson Education.

15

Conditions Affecting Fetal Growth

Fetal growth in utero can be affected by a variety of maternal, fetal, placental, and environmental conditions. Some conditions result in low birth weight, whereas others result in macrosomia, which has different, but still significant implications. Monitoring for causative factors and signs and symptoms during pregnancy can alert the neonatal team to potential variations in fetal growth that impact the neonatal period.

During this part of the orientation, the nurse will be able to:

1. Differentiate between the different categories within the low birth weight definition.
2. Describe the difference between intrauterine growth restriction and small for gestational age.
3. Identify risk factors for macrosomia.
4. Detail adverse events associated with post-maturity.

LOW BIRTH WEIGHT

Low birth weight (LBW)	Birth weight of a live-born infant less than 2,500 g (5.5 lbs), regardless of gestational age
Very low birth weight (VLBW)	Birth weight of a live-born infant less than 1,500 g (3.3 lbs)
Extremely low birth weight (ELBW)	Birth weight of a live-born infant less than 1,000 g (2.2 lbs)

Etiological/Risk Factors

- Small parental stature/familial inheritance
- Congenital defects
- Chromosomal disorders
- Multiparity
- Previous LBW infants
- Poor nutrition
- Maternal heart disease
- Maternal hypertension
- Smoking
- Drug addiction
- Alcohol abuse
- Lead exposure
- Insufficient prenatal care

Adverse Effects

- Birth asphyxia
- Meconium aspiration
- Unstable blood sugar levels
- Developmental delays
- Psychological adjustment issues
- Intellectual disability
- Developmental delays

Nursing Considerations for LBW Infants

- Monitor weight loss/gain in newborn period.
- Feed frequently.
- Assess for respiratory problems, poor postnatal growth, and infections.
- Educate parents that LBW infants are more at risk for chronic health issues.
- Closely monitor the achievement of developmental milestones during infancy due to an increased risk of neurodevelopmental delays.
- Refer for parenting interventions as appropriate.

INTRAUTERINE GROWTH RESTRICTION

Intrauterine growth restriction (IUGR) is an alteration in fetal growth in which the fetus's/newborn's weight is at or below the tenth percentile. Infants within the third percentile are at the highest risk for perinatal outcomes, including fetal/neonatal death. IUGR typically results from alterations in placental functioning during pregnancy.

Symmetrical IUGR occurs when both head and body growth are symmetrically small, and represents 20% to 30% of all IUGR. It typically begins in the first or second trimester and is associated with poorer clinical outcomes (Davidson, Ladewig, & London, 2020).

Asymmetrical IUGR occurs when the body is proportionally smaller than the head during growth. The majority of IUGRs (7% to 80%) involve asymmetry, which typically begins in the third trimester and is associated with better clinical outcomes (Davidson et al., 2020).

Small for gestational age (SGA) refers to an infant who is less than the tenth percentile for birth weight. *Very small for gestational age* refers to two standard deviations below the population norm or at less than the third percentile (Davidson et al., 2020).

Etiological/Risk Factors

- Preeclampsia/eclampsia
- Multiple gestation
- Placental abnormalities
- Living in high altitudes
- Congenital/chromosomal abnormalities
- Alcohol abuse
- Maternal obesity
- Clotting disorders
- Substance abuse
- Hypertension
- Heart disease
- Kidney disease
- Poor nutrition
- Smoking
- Diabetes in pregnancy, including gestational diabetes
- Anemia
- Thrombophilia

Adverse Effects

- Nonreassuring fetal status in labor
- Need for cesarean delivery
- Intraventricular hemorrhage
- Periventricular leukomalacia
- Hypoxic ischemic encephalopathy
- Necrotizing enterocolitis
- Bronchopulmonary dysplasia

- Sepsis
- Perinatal mortality

Nursing Considerations for Infants With IUGR

- Ensure that the neonatal resuscitation team is present for delivery.
- Maintain thermoregulation.
- Stabilize newborn.
- Monitor labs since newborn is at risk for:

  - Hypoglycemia
  - Hypocalcemia
  - Polycythemia
  - Hyperbilirubinemia

- Screen for congenital anomalies.
- Screen for congenital infection.
- Specialized NICU care may be needed.

LARGE FOR GESTATIONAL AGE AND INFANTS WITH MACROSOMIA

Large-for-gestational-age (LGA) newborns are defined as newborns born at or above the ninetieth percentile for gestational age. Approximately 9% of all births are classified as LGA, with Native Americans having the highest rates (Davidson et al., 2020). *Macrosomia* refers to excessive intrauterine growth beyond a specific threshold regardless of gestational age. The incidence of macrosomia is 10% (Davidson et al., 2020). This condition is usually defined as a birth weight of greater than 4,000 or 4,500 g.

Etiological/Risk Factors

- Postdate pregnancy
- Gestational diabetes
- Preexisting maternal diabetes
- Male newborn
- Genetic predisposition
- Maternal obesity
- Excessive maternal weight gain in pregnancy
- Multiparity
- Congenital anomalies
- Hydrops fetalis
- Erythroblastosis fetalis

- Use of some antibiotics (amoxicillin, pivampicillin) during pregnancy
- Genetic disorders associated with excessive fetal growth

  - Beckwith-Wiedemann syndrome
  - Sotos syndrome

Adverse Effects

- Birth trauma
- Shoulder dystocia
- Facial bruising
- Scalp contusions
- Brachial plexus injuries
- Operative vaginal birth
- Cesarean delivery
- Hypoglycemia
- Poor motor skills
- Feeding difficulties
- Irritability
- Difficult to arouse
- Polycythemia
- Hyperviscosity
- Hypocalcemia
- Jaundice
- Respiratory distress
- Erb's palsy
- Increased morbidity and mortality
- Increased risks of childhood leukemia, Wilms' tumor, and osteosarcoma

Nursing Considerations for LGA Infants and Infants With Macrosomia

- Have a neonatal resuscitation team present at delivery.
- Anticipate possible shoulder dystocia.
- Anticipate the possible need for cesarean birth.
- Complete a gestational age assessment.
- Monitor for hypoglycemia immediately following birth.
- Prevent cold stress.
- Obtain CBC and chemistry panel.
- Assess for injuries associated with birth trauma.
- Reassure parents that bruising is temporary.
- When injuries are present, obtain a referral for appropriate treatment and follow-up.

The most common cause of macrosomia is maternal diabetes. Infants who are born LGA are at a higher risk of developing diabetes later in life.

POSTTERM NEWBORNS

Postterm pregnancy (also known as postmature or prolonged pregnancy) refers to the gestation period of more than 42 weeks. Its incidence is 3% to 12% (Davidson et al., 2020).

Postdate pregnancy refers to a gestation period continued after the expected date of confinement has passed.

Etiological/Risk Factors

- Primiparity
- Prior postterm pregnancy
- Male fetus
- Family history
- Genetic factors

Adverse Effects

- Uteroplacental insufficiency
- Prolonged labor
- Cephalopelvic disproportion
- Shoulder dystocia
- Nonreassuring fetal status on labor
- Increased cesarean delivery
- Orthopedic injuries at birth
- Neurological injuries at birth
- Meconium and meconium aspiration
- Neonatal acidemia
- Low Apgar scores
- Macrosomia
- Hypoglycemia
- Polycythemia
- Fetal dysmaturity syndrome (postmaturity syndrome)
- Neonatal morbidity and mortality
- Stillbirth (six times more likely in postterm pregnancies)
- Sudden infant death syndrome
- Infant death in first year of life

Nursing Considerations for Postterm Newborns

- Have a neonatal resuscitation team present at delivery.
- Anticipate possible shoulder dystocia.
- Anticipate the possible need for a cesarean birth.
- Provide a physical exam to assess for birth injury.
- Obtain a referral to a specialist if an injury occurred during birth.
- Maintain thermoregulation since cold stress is common.
- Assess for congenital defects.
- Monitor for seizures or other signs of neurological injury.
- Monitor respiratory status, since respiratory issues can occur in the first 24 hours.
- Monitor labs for hypoglycemia and polycythemia.

References

Davidson, M. R., Ladewig, P. L., & London, M. L. (2020). *Old's maternal newborn nursing and women's health across the lifespan* (11th ed.). Boston, MA: Pearson Education.

16

Hematological Disorders

Hematological disorders in the newborn may include inherited or acquired conditions. Newborn screening can provide important clinical information that guides the care of the newborn with a hematological disorder. Ongoing assessment is needed to identify the newborn and ensure the condition is adequately treated to prevent adverse outcomes.

During this part of the orientation, the nurse will be able to:

1. Compare and contrast inherited and acquired hematological conditions in the newborn.
2. List common hemorrhagic disease that may be present in the newborn period
3. Discuss the differences between early and late-onset thrombocytopenia in the newborn period.
4. Examine the different types of inherited hemolytic anemias.
5. Detail strategies for interventions for the newborn with disseminated intravascular coagulation (DIC).

HEMATOLOGICAL DISORDERS (HRC)

Hematological disorders encountered in the newborn period include inherited clotting deficiencies (factor VIII deficiency) or acquired disorders, such as hemorrhagic disease, thrombocytopenia, newborn anemia, disseminated intravascular coagulation (DIC), and liver failure.

Nursing Considerations

- Obtain pregnancy, labor, and birth history.
- Obtain family history of genetic hematological disorders.
- Obtain parental ethnic group to determine risk factors for inherited disorders.
- Provide laboratory testing to determine the type of hematological disorder.
- Provide immediate treatment to correct the disorder.
- Administer medications or blood products.

Hemorrhagic Disease in the Newborn

Hemorrhagic disease in the newborn infant is caused by the deficiency of the vitamin K-dependent clotting factors (II, VII, IX, and X) and occurs in 0.25% to 1.7% of newborns who have not received vitamin K administration after birth. In newborns with hemorrhagic disease:

- Vitamin K was typically not given after birth.
- Bleeding occurs within 5 days to 6 weeks.
- Bleeding sites may include the gastrointestinal tract, umbilical cord, circumcision site, and nose.
- Risk for intracranial hemorrhage
- Increased risk in infants of mothers taking hydantoin anticonvulsants or warfarin
- Increased incidence in breastfed infants
- DIC and hepatic failure must be ruled out.
- Intravenous vitamin K is administered; injections are contraindicated.

Fast Fact

Any infant that shows any signs of bleeding during the newborn period warrants immediate evaluation for liver or bleeding disorders.

THROMBOCYTOPENIA

Thrombocytopenia is defined as a platelet count under 150,000/µL (usually less than 50,000/µL, may be less than 10,000/µL). It can be idiopathic or related to a deficiency of clotting factors. Newborns affected by Rh isoimmunization are at risk for isoimmune thrombocytopenia. The most common cause occurs in term neonates and is associated with placental insufficiency, which typically resolves 10 days after birth. Preterm thrombocytopenia is commonly associated with NEC or sepsis and requires aggressive management. The management varies with whether the onset occurs within the first 72 hours of birth or after 72 hours of life. Table 16.1 reviews the management of thrombocytopenia.

Table 16.1

Management of Thrombocytopenia in Neonates

Type of Thrombocytopenia (TCP)	Lab Values	Nursing Considerations
Early Onset (Within 72 hours after birth)	Mild to moderate (PC 50,000–149,000/µL) Severe (PC < 50,000)	If the baby is well with no evidence of sepsis or placenta insufficiency, monitor to ensure PLT is rising or within normal range. If the baby has been subjected to placental insufficiency and appears ill, monitor for sepsis and DIC. If TCP persists, consider thrombocytopenia-absent radius, amegakaryocytic thrombocytopenia with radioulnar synostosis, or Fanconi anemia. Assess for genetic disorders. Assess for maternal TCP; assess for the presence splenomegaly and hepatomegaly, which may indicate a viral etiology. Viral screening should include TORCH infections, HIV, and enterovirus. Screen for thrombosis and congenital thrombocytopenia.
Late Onset (Occurs 72 hours or later after birth)		Screen for bacterial or fungal sepsis and NEC. If sepsis or NEC and PC is normalizing with treatment regimen, then no further evaluation is warranted. If sepsis and NEC are ruled out, a clinical evaluation for other disorders is warranted: DIC, viral infection, thrombosis, drug-induced TCP, inborn errors of metabolism, or Fanconi anemia.

In newborns with thrombocytopenia:

- Screen for neonatal alloimmune thrombocytopenia if it is severe and occurs within 24 hours of birth.
- Transfusion is necessary for term newborn if the total platelet count is lower than 20,000/μL or active bleeding is present.
- Transfusion is necessary for the preterm infant if there is a risk for intraventricular hemorrhage or if the total platelet count is lower than 40,000/μL.
- Isoimmune thrombocytopenia requires transfusions with maternal platelets until platelet counts reach 50,000/μL or higher.
- Newborns of mothers who have idiopathic thrombocytopenic purpura do not typically need treatment; if bleeding occurs, prednisone 2 mg/kg/day is given for 7 to 14 days.

NEWBORN ANEMIA

Anemia can occur as a result of hemorrhage, hemolysis, or failure to produce red blood cells. Newborn hemorrhage can occur as a result of:

- In utero etiologies (fetoplacental and fetomaternal)
- Perinatal etiologies (cord rupture, placenta previa, placenta abruption)
- After birth (intracranial hemorrhage, cephalohematoma, ruptured liver or spleen)

Hemolysis, which is almost always associated with hyperbilirubinemia, can occur as a result of multiple etiologies, including:

- Blood group incompatibilities
- Enzyme abnormalities
- Membrane abnormalities
- Infection
- DIC

POLYCYTHEMIA

Polycythemia is categorized by a capillary hematocrit that is greater than 68% or a venous hematocrit greater than 65%. In newborns with polycythemia, hyperviscosity with decreased perfusion of the capillary beds occurs. Polycythemia occurs in 2% to 5% of all live births and occurs more commonly in newborns who are small for gestational age or large for gestational age (Davidson, Ladewig, & London, 2020). Common etiologies include:

- Twin–twin transfusion
- Maternal–fetal transfusion

- Intrapartum transfusion from the placenta
- Chronic intrauterine hypoxia

Treatment is warranted for all symptomatic infants. Treatment for symptomatic newborns varies. The recommended treatment includes:

- Isovolumic partial exchange transfusion with 5% albumin or normal saline
- Blood withdrawl from the umbilical artery while the infusion is administered over 15 to 30 minutes
- Obtaining a desired hematocrit value of 50% to 55%
- Obtaining a blood volume of 80 mL/kg

INHERITED HEMOLYTIC ANEMIAS

Inherited hemolytic anemias are associated with genetic defects that control red blood cell production (Table 16.2).

Table 16.2

Types of Inherited Hemolytic Anemias		
Type of Inherited Anemia	**Abnormality**	**Population(s) At Greatest Risk**
Sickle cell anemia	Abnormally shaped hemoglobin, which are sickle- or crescent-shaped and have decreased oxygen-carrying capabilities	African Americans
	Red blood cells have a shorter life span. Bone marrow cannot make enough red blood cells to meet needs.	
Thalassemia	Decreased hemoglobin levels—this causes the body to make fewer healthy red blood cells than normal.	People of Southeast Asian, Indian, Chinese, Filipino, Mediterranean, or African origin or descent
Hereditary spherocytosis	Defect in the surface membrane of red blood cells causes them to have a spherical or ball-like shape. These blood cells have a life span that is shorter than normal.	Northern European descent

(continued)

Table 16.2

Types of Inherited Hemolytic Anemias (*continued*)

Type of Inherited Anemia	Abnormality	Population(s) At Greatest Risk
Hereditary elliptocytosis (ovalocytosis)	Cell membrane abnormality in which the red blood cells are elliptic (oval) in shape. They are not as flexible as normal red blood cells, and they have a shorter life span.	
Glucose-6-phosphate dehydrogenase (G6PD) deficiency	Lack of G6PD enzyme results in red blood cells rupturing when they come into contact with certain substances in the bloodstream.	Males of African or Mediterranean descent; African American males
Pyruvate kinase deficiency	Lack of pyruvate kinase causes early cell death and breakdown.	Amish

DISSEMINATED INTRAVASCULAR COAGULATION

DIC is a condition of uncontrolled bleeding that occurs with simultaneous, uncontrolled clotting, which occurs when inappropriate activation and consumption of clotting factors result in a hemorrhagic state because of inadequate hemostasis (Eichenwald, Hansen, Martin, & Stark, 2017).

The most common etiologies include:

- Asphyxia
- Hypoxemia
- Shock
- Acidosis
- Sepsis
- Respiratory distress syndrome
- Hyaline membrane disease

Adverse Effects and Consequences of DIC

- Uncontrolled bleeding

  - Petechiae
  - Purpura
  - Ecchymoses
  - Hematomas

- Ischemic damage
- Organ failure
- Death

Treatment Strategies for DIC

- Monitor laboratory values for progression of the disorder.
- Identify and correct the underlying cause.
- Administer antibiotics if infection present.
- Administer transfusions of platelets and/or fresh frozen plasma.
- Administer transfusions of packed red blood cells to correct anemia.
- Provide ventilator assistance.
- Administer vasopressor drips.
- Monitor vital signs.
- Monitor fluid and electrolyte balance.
- Provide nutritional support.
- Avoid venipuncture and invasive procedures.

References

Davidson, M. R., Ladewig, P. L., & London, M. L. (2020). *Old's maternal newborn nursing and women's health across the lifespan* (11th ed.). Boston, MA: Pearson Education.

Eichenwald, E. C., Hansen, A. R., Martin, C. R., & Stark, A. R. (2017). *Cloherty and Stark's manual of neonatal care* (8th ed.). Philadelphia, PA: Wolters Kluwer.

17

Conditions Associated With Maternal Risk

Certain medical conditions present during pregnancy or at the time of birth may put the neonate at an increased risk for adverse outcomes. Infections, maternal diabetes, and substance abuse can negatively impact the newborn at the time of birth and in the newborn period. These conditions warrant prompt intervention and ongoing assessment in order to provide the best treatment modalities for the newborn.

During this part of the orientation, the nurse will be able to:

1. Identify common maternal infections and their adverse outcomes that the newborn may experience.
2. Detail appropriate treatments for the most commonly occurring maternal infections.
3. Discuss potential neonatal adverse effects associated with maternal gestational diabetes.
4. Differentiate the different fetal alcohol syndrome disorders.
5. Discuss adverse outcomes that may occur with substance abuse in the newborn.
6. Outline the various screening tools used to assess for neonatal abstinence syndrome.

NEWBORNS EXPOSED TO MATERNAL INFECTION

Fetuses exposed to infections in utero have a potential to acquire the infection through vertical transmission or during a vaginal birth from the mother. Some infections carry more potential for adverse outcomes than others.

Cytomegalovirus (CMV)

Adverse Outcomes

- Prematurity
- Intrauterine growth restriction
- Jaundice
- Hepatosplenomegaly
- Periventricular calcifications
- Chorioretinitis
- Pneumonitis
- Hepatitis
- Sensorineural hearing loss
- Intellectual disability
- Visual disturbances

Treatment

- Diagnosis is made by viral culture of saliva, urine or tissue or PCR using saliva, urine, blood, or tissue.
- Urine and saliva have greatest sensitivity and are present first 3 weeks following birth.
- Treat with ganciclour or valganciclovir.

Herpes Simplex Virus (HSV)

Adverse Outcomes

- Local or systemic disease can occur between 1 to4 weeks after birth and may include localized lesions.

Treatment

- Diagnosis is made via a viral culture or HSV PCR or lesion scrapings.
- Intravenous acyclovir is given for 21 days for systemic disease or for 14 days for skin lesions. Eye lesions require topical trifluridine.
- Supportive therapy includes IVF, respiratory support, and assessment and treatment of clotting abnormalities and seizures.

Rubella

Adverse Outcomes

- Disease occurs in newborns when the mother is infected during the first 16 weeks of pregnancy, when the most adverse outcomes are likely to occur.

  - IUGR
  - Microcephaly
  - Meningoencephalitis
  - Cataracts
  - Hearing loss
  - Bone abnormalities
  - Hepatosplenomegaly
  - Cardiac defects

- Additional complications

  - Thrombocytopenia
  - Dermal erythropoiesis
  - Adenopathy hemolytic anemia
  - Pneumonia

Treatment

- Prevention of infection and viral exposure during pregnancy is key. Treatment is based on addressing the adverse outcomes associated with the infection.
- If suspected disease, viral titers should be drawn. Persistent titers beyond 6 to 12 months suggest congenital disease.
- Assess for hearing loss, intellectual disability, abnormal behavior, endocrinopathies, and progressive encephalitis.

Toxoplasmosis

Adverse Outcomes

- Preterm birth
- IUGR
- Jaundice
- Hepatosplenomegaly
- Myocarditis
- Pneumonitis
- Rash
- Chorioretinitis
- Hydrocephalus

- Intracranial calcifications
- Microcephaly
- Seizures

Treatment

- Diagnosis is made by amniotic fluid PCR, serological testing, brain imagining, CSF analysis, eye examination, and PCR testing.
- Treatments are pyrimethamine, sulfadiazine, or leucovorin.
- Long-term effects can include ongoing neurological sequela or early death.

Hepatitis B

Adverse Outcomes

- Jaundice
- Lethargy
- Failure to thrive
- Abdominal distention
- Clay-colored stools
- Acute liver failure
- Low birth weight
- Hepatomegaly
- Ascites
- Hyperbilirubinemia
- Chronic hepatitis
- Cirrhosis
- Severe liver disease
- Hepatocellular cancer
- Most infants are asymptomatic but can develop an asymptomatic infection.

Treatment

- Diagnosis is made by serological testing.
- Treatment may include interferon alfa, lamivudine, or adefovir.
- Mothers who are HBsAg-positive should get one dose of HBIG 0.5 mL within the first 12 hours of birth. Also, infants should receive recombinant HBV vaccination with a three vaccination schedule.

Syphilis

Adverse Outcomes

- Skin lesions
- Lymphadenopathy
- Hepatosplenomegaly

- Failure to thrive
- Blood-tinged nasal discharge
- Perioral fissures
- Meningitis
- Choroiditis
- Hydrocephalus
- Seizures
- Intellectual disability
- Osteochondritis
- Pseudo-paralysis
- Early congenital syphilis occurs within the first 3 months with symptoms of papular rash on mouth, nose, diaper area, soles of feet, and palms of hands. Nasal congestion is common. Osteochondritis occurs within the first 8 months.

Treatment

- Testing includes RPR, VDRL, and lumbar puncture with CSF analysis.
- Titers in infants should be obtained every 2 to 3 months until negative or four-fold decline is noted.
- Treatment is crystalline PCN G 50,000 units/kg IV q 12 hours for 7 days then q 8 hours for 3 days or Procaine PCN G 50,000 units/kg IM daily for 10 days. If a day is missed, the series needs to be restarted.
- In women treated in pregnancy, a single dose of Benzathine PCN 50,000 units/kg IM / one is given.

Listeriosis

Adverse Outcomes

- May become infected in utero or at the time of birth via vaginal secretions
- Granuloma formation on skin, liver, adrenal glands, lymphatic tissue, lungs, and brain may occur. Skin lesions are known as granulomatosis infantsepticum.
- Can result in respiratory distress, shock, and death in the immediate neonatal period. Preterm birth, stillbirth, neonatal sepsis, LBW, circulation and respiratory collapse, meningitis, and sepsis may also occur.

Treatment

- Diagnosis includes cultures of blood, gastric aspirate, meconium, or infected tissue.
- Treatment consists of ampicillin with aminoglycoside in a 14-day course.

Chlamydia

Adverse Outcomes

- Newborns are at risk for infection from contamination in the birth canal.
- 1-to-3-week incubation period
- Conjunctivitis can result in eye redness, swelling, and discharge. Pneumonia can also occur characterized by cough and tachypnea.

Treatment

- Preventative treatment is required by state law in the United States.
- Erythromycin 0.5% ophthalmic ointment is administered as a thin strip 0.5 to 1 cm long starting at the inner canthus and is spread to the entire eye when the eye is closed.
- Women with a positive chlamydia culture are treated immediately during pregnancy with azithromycin 1 g in a single dose.
- Other effective treatments include doxycycline, erythromycin, ofloxacin, or levofloxacin.

Gonorrhea

Adverse Outcomes

- Newborns at risk for infection from contamination in the birth canal.
- 2-to-4-day incubation period
- Conjunctivitis can result in eye redness, swelling, and purulent discharge. Adverse outcomes may include sepsis and meningitis.

Treatment

- Preventative treatment is required by state law in the United States.
- Erythromycin 0.5% ophthalmic ointment is administered as a thin strip 0.5 to 1 cm long starting at the inner canthus and is spread to the entire eye when the eye is closed.
- Women who test positive prior to the onset of labor should be treated with ceftriaxone 250 mg IM and azithromycin 1 g orally or, alternatively, cefixime 400 mg po and azithromycin 1 g orally.

NEWBORNS OF DIABETIC MOTHERS

Newborns of diabetic mothers may be born to women with gestational, type 1, or type 2 diabetes. Approximately 3% to 9% of infants are classified as infants of diabetic mothers. Only 8% of women who have abnormal glucose regulation during pregnancy have type 2 diabetes. Type 1 diabetes in pregnancy accounts for only 1% of all women with diabetes in pregnancy, with 92% of diabetic pregnant women having gestational diabetes (Davidson, Ladewig, & London, 2020).

Etiological/Risk Factors

- Family history
- Native American, Black, Hispanic, and Asian race
- Maternal obesity

Adverse Effects

- Birth injury
- Cesarean birth
- Birth defects
- Increased NICU admission rates
- Hypoglycemia
- LGA
- SGA
- Macrosomia
- Increased neonatal morbidity and mortality
- Childhood glucose intolerance
- Elevated serum insulin levels in childhood
- Childhood metabolic syndrome
- Long-term cardiovascular risks
- Neurocognitive disorders (attention deficit hyperactivity disorder, altered neurobehavioral functioning)

Nursing Considerations

- Have neonatal resuscitation team present at delivery.
- Anticipate possible shoulder dystocia.
- Anticipate possible need for a cesarean birth.
- Evaluate respiratory status.
- Provide respiratory intervention as needed.
- Provide physical exam to assess for birth injury and congenital defects.
- Obtain a heel stick for glucose testing within 4 hours of birth.
- Monitor for cold stress and temperature instability.
- Provide continuous blood glucose monitoring (every 4 hours per institution protocol).
- Monitor labs for hypoglycemia, hyperbilirubinemia, and hypocalcemia.
- Provide parental education to reduce risk of childhood obesity and lifelong complications.
- Encourage breastfeeding in this population.

Approximately one-third of women with gestational diabetes will develop overt diabetes within 5 years of delivery.

NEWBORNS EXPOSED TO SUBSTANCE ABUSE, ALCOHOL, AND TOBACCO (HRC)

Substance abuse in pregnancy can create adverse maternal, fetal, and neonatal outcomes. A comprehensive review is needed to determine whether there is any history of a substance abuse problem/disorder and, whether so, the mother's previous drug-use patterns. Prenatal, labor, and birth history should also be obtained. It is important to elicit information in a nonthreatening, nonjudgmental way.

Alcohol Use in Pregnancy

Alcohol use continues in 7.6% of pregnant women, with 12.2% of pregnant women consuming at least one alcohol-containing beverage within the last 30 days. Of those women who continually use alcohol during pregnancy, 1.4% are classified as binge drinkers (drinking more than six drinks on one occasion). Of women who binge drink in pregnancy, the average frequency of episodes was three times per month.

- Aged 35 to 44 years (14.3%)
- White (8.3%)
- College graduate (10.0%)
- Unmarried (13.4%)
- Employed (9.6%)

The strongest predictor for alcohol use in pregnancy is past use prior to conception. A detailed history of alcohol use patterns prior to pregnancy can determine the risk of use and continuation during the prenatal period.

FETAL ALCOHOL SPECTRUM DISORDERS

Fetal alcohol spectrum disorders (FASDs) are a group of conditions that can occur in a person who is exposed to alcohol in utero. The effects of alcohol consumption may include physical alterations and behavioral or learning disorders.

Fetal Alcohol Syndrome

Fetal alcohol syndrome (FAS) is the most severe disorder on the FASD spectrum and often results in fetal death. FAS is associated with a combination of the following (Eichenwald, Hansen, Martin, & Stark, 2017):

- Abnormal facial features
- Growth problems
- Central nervous system issues
- Learning, memory, attention span, and communication deficits
- Vision problems
- Hearing loss
- Difficulty interacting with others

Alcohol-Related Neurodevelopmental Disorder

Alcohol-related neurodevelopmental disorder commonly results in a variety of impairments, including:
- Intellectual disabilities
- Behavioral problems
- Learning disabilities
- Poor school performance with:

  - Math
  - Memory
  - Attention
  - Judgment
  - Poor impulse control

Alcohol-Related Birth Defects

People with alcohol-related birth defects have birth defects that include:

- Vision or hearing problems
- Cardiac defects
- Impairment of kidneys
- Skeletal disorders

SUBSTANCE ABUSE IN PREGNANCY

Approximately 4% of pregnant women are drug dependent during pregnancy. Commonly used substances include marijuana, cocaine, ecstasy and other amphetamines, and heroin. Substance abuse in pregnancy has been associated with adverse fetal and newborn outcomes. Tobacco use in pregnancy continues in 10.4% of pregnancies. The adverse effects vary depending on the type of substance used (Forray, 2016).

Marijuana

Incidence: 12%

Short-Term Effects

- Low birth weight and shortened fetal length
- Preterm labor and preterm birth
- Admission to intensive care unit
- Stillbirth

Long-Term Effects

- Infants are more likely to have developmental and speech delays and learning and behavioral issues.
- Abnormal childhood and adolescent brain growth
- Abnormalities with executive function, attention problems, poor academic achievement, and increased behavioral issues in childhood and adolescence
- Developmental deficits in childhood, greater addiction risk in adolescence
- Adolescence with reduced ability to self-regulate, focus, and poorer memory

Cocaine

Incidence: 0.3%–1.0%

Short-Term Effects

- Premature rupture of membranes
- Placental abruption
- Preterm labor and preterm birth
- Low birth weight and small-for-gestational-age infants; smaller-than-normal head circumference
- With hemorrhage, fetal distress and fetal death can occur.

Long-Term Effects

- Neonatal withdraw may occur.
- Possible language, motor, and cognitive development
- Poorer self-regulation, focus, attention, and memory
- Higher incidence of birth defects (genitals, kidney, brain, urinary tract)
- Cerebral palsy

Methamphetamines

Incidence: 0.7% to 4.8%

Short-Term Effects

- Small-for-gestational-age and shorter gestational ages; lower birth weight and small head circumference
- Inadequate prenatal care
- Multiple substance drug use
- Preterm birth
- Fetal loss
- Preeclampsia
- Placental abnormalties
- Gestational hypertension
- Cesarean birth
- NICU admission
- Intrauterine fetal death

Long-Term Effects

- Developmental and behavioral defects
- Club foot
- Cleft lip/palate
- Heart defects

Opioid Use

Incidence: 0.6%

Short-Term Effects

- Chorioamnionitis
- SIDS
- Premature rupture of the membranes
- Meconium staining
- Preeclampsia
- Placental abruption

- Low birth weight
- Respiratory problems
- Third trimester bleeding
- Toxemia
- Perinatal mortality

Long-Term Effects

- Neonatal abstinence syndrome (NAS), whereby opiate exposure in utero triggers a postnatal withdrawal syndrome
- Irritability
- Feeding difficulties
- Tremors
- Hypertonia
- Emesis
- Loose stools
- Seizures
- Respiratory distress
- Increased hospitalization and healthcare utilization costs
- Postnatal growth deficiency
- Microcephaly
- Neurobehavioral problems

Common Club Drugs (Phenylcyclidine [PCP/Angel Dust], Ketamine [Special K], And Lysergic Acid Diethylamide [LSD/Acid])

Incidence: Unknown

Short-Term Effects

- Low birth weight
- Hypotonia
- Microcephaly
- Facial defects and facial asymmetry
- Intrauterine growth restriction
- Preterm birth
- Fetal loss

Long-Term Effects

- Ocular defects
- NAS
- Neurological deficits
- Behavioral problems
- Learning disabilities

Glue and Solvent Use

Incidence: Unknown

Short-Term Effects

- Spontaneous abortion
- Premature birth
- Intrauterine growth restriction
- Small for gestational age

Long-Term Effects

- Congenital malformations
- Craniofacial defects
- Growth abnormalities in childhood
- Deficits in cognitive, speech, and motor skills
- Neurodevelopmental delays
- Skeletal abnormalities

Heroin

Incidence: Estimated 20,000 neonates annually

Short-Term Effects

- Premature birth
- Low birth weight
- Premature rupture of membranes
- Intrauterine growth restriction
- Breathing difficulties
- Low blood sugar (hypoglycemia)
- Bleeding within the brain (intracranial hemorrhage)
- Infant death

Long-Term Effects

- NAS
- Higher incidence of HIV infection.
- Feeding difficulties and sleep irregularities.
- Congenital birth defects (heart, spine, eyes)
- SIDS
- Learning disabilities and behavioral disturbances.

Tobacco Use in Pregnancy

Tobacco use in pregnancy is contraindicated and has been associated
with adverse effects on the pregnancy and developing fetus. Pregnant

women should be counseled to discontinue smoking during pregnancy and to avoid second-hand smoke. Tobacco use in pregnancy is associated with (Wilson & Thorp, 2008):

- Small for gestational age
- Preterm birth
- Placental disorders
- Low birth weight
- SIDS
- Cleft lip/cleft palate
- SIDS

Neonatal Abstinence Syndrome

NAS describes a group of problems that occur in newborns who have been exposed to addictive illegal or prescription drugs in utero. Babies of mothers who consume alcohol during pregnancy may have a similar condition. These infants continue to have risks for adverse health outcomes that continue in the neonatal period and during the first year of life, with some having lifelong adverse health conditions and implications. Due to the psychosocial factors associated with substance abuse, multiple concerns exist in the newborn period, including:

- Alterations in infant–parent attachment
- Newborn safety issues
- Exposure to secondhand smoke
- Infant mental health issues
- Exposure to domestic violence

Treatment Measures for Infants With NAS

Tests that may be done to diagnose withdrawal in a newborn include:

- The recommended treatment is based on the type of drug used, infant's overall health and transition, and gestational age at the time of birth.
- NAS scoring assessment should be performed, which assigns points based on each symptom and its severity and helps determine treatment course.
- Toxicology screen of first bowel movements (meconium)
- Drug screening via urinalysis
- Some infants may require medication for withdrawal.
- High-calorie formula may be needed.

References

Davidson, M. R., Ladewig, P. L., & London, M. L. (2020). *Old's maternal newborn nursing and women's health across the lifespan* (11th ed.). Boston, MA: Pearson Education.

Eichenwald, E. C., Hansen, A. R., Martin, C. R., & Stark, A. R. (2017). *Cloherty and Stark's manual of neonatal care* (8th ed.). Philadelphia, PA: Wolters Kluwer.

Forray, A. (2016). Substance abuse in pregnancy. *Faculty Review, 5*, F1000, 887. doi:10.12688/f1000research.7645.1

Wilson, J. K., & Thorp, J. M. (2008). Substance abuse in pregnancy. *Journal of Global Library of Women's Medicine*. doi:10.3843/GLOWM.10115

VI

Genetic and Congenital Disorders

18

Genetic and Congenital Disorders

The birth of a baby is typically seen as a happy event, with the expectation that the newborn will be healthy. Although some parents will know beforehand of a potential birth defect, others may become aware of their newborn's medical complications only after delivery. When a baby is born with a genetic or congenital defect or when an unexpected birth outcome occurs, parents are often devastated and in need of intense psychosocial support and education. The nurse plays a key role in providing education about the newborn's condition, short- and long-term care needs, and referrals for immediate and long-term, community-based support services for the family.

During this part of the orientation, the nurse will be able to:

1. Describe the most common types of birth disorders.
2. Identify possible etiological factors for specific birth disorders.
3. Discuss possible complications that may occur as a result of specific birth disorders.

INTRODUCTION OF PREFERRED DISABILITY LANGUAGE

When referring to certain medical conditions or individuals with specific disabilities, use appropriate language. Specific disability language should be used when discussing specific conditions when relevant to identify the presence of a disability. This is often the case in a medical or healthcare setting. Avoid words such as "abnormal" or "unhealthy," and slang terms. "Disability" is appropriate and should be used.

Do not use less correct terms, including (National Youth Leadership Network, 2020):

- Handicapped
- Differently-abled
- Cripple or crippled
- Victim
- Retarded
- Stricken
- Poor
- Unfortunate
- Special needs

GENETIC AND CONGENITAL DISORDERS

Genetic disorders (also known as genetic defects) are heritable abnormalities passed down from the genome or occur with new mutations in the DNA. "Genetic disorder" is the broad term for any defect resulting from a genetic-related etiology. The different types of genetic disorders can be inherited in a number of ways.

Congenital defects are those that are present at birth.

Chromosomal abnormalities are large-scale duplications or deletions of chromosomal segments or entire chromosomes that result in birth defects. The most common chromosomal disorder is Down syndrome, which occurs in 1 in 800 births (Davidson, Ladewig, & London, 2020).

Mendelian disorders (single-gene disorders) occur as the result of a mutation to a single gene. It is estimated there are over 10,000 single-gene mutation disorders. The most common is hypercholesterolemia, which has an incidence of 5% (Davidson et al., 2020). The different modes of genetic inheritance are listed in Table 18.1.

Multifactorial inheritance disorders occur as a result of interaction between multiple genes and environments. In multifactorial disorders:

- Malformations can be mild to severe.
- In more severe cases, a greater number of genes are typically involved.
- Some disorders are more common in one gender than in the other.

- If a condition occurs that is rare for that gender, a greater number of genes are likely involved.
- When a defect is present in close family members, risk of occurrence is higher.
- When multiple family members have the same defect, risk of occurrence increases.
- Once a specific defect occurs in one pregnancy, risk of reoccurrence is higher in subsequent pregnancies.

Table 18.1

Different Types of Genetic Disorders		
Type of Genetic Disorder	**Description of Disorder**	**Examples of Disorders**
Autosomal dominant	Only one mutated copy of the gene is necessary for a person to be affected. The affected gene overshadows the normal gene. Typically, a parent is affected with the disorder. Males and females are equally affected. Incidence of inheritance is 50%.	Huntington's disease Hereditary nonpolyposis colorectal cancer Neurofibromatosis types 1 and 2 Phocomelia
Autosomal recessive	Two copies of the abnormal gene must be present. An affected person usually has unaffected parents (carriers) who each carry a single copy of the mutated gene. Risk of inheritance with disease is 25%. When both parents are carriers, there is a 25% chance the child will be a carrier. Males and females are equally affected.	Cystic fibrosis Sickle-cell disease Tay–Sachs disease Phenylketonuria Galactosemia
X-linked dominant	Caused by mutations in genes on the X chromosome. Although it is extremely rare, females and males can inherit this, but males are more severely affected. When the father is the carrier, male offspring are not affected; however, the female offspring would be. (I.e., there is no male-to-male inheritance.) When the woman is the carrier, 50% of offspring are affected.	X-linked hypophosphatemic rickets Rett's syndrome Klinefelter syndrome

(*continued*)

Table 18.1

Different Types of Genetic Disorders (*continued*)		
Type of Genetic Disorder	**Description of Disorder**	**Examples of Disorders**
X-linked recessive	Caused by mutations in genes on the X chromosome that are manifested by the male, who is the carrier of the abnormal gene, via the female line. Men are more commonly affected. Carrier mothers will affect 50% of male offspring, and 50% of female offspring will become carriers. Fathers cannot pass on the disorder to male offspring, but all female offspring will become carriers.	Hemophilia A Duchenne muscular dystrophy Lesch-Nyhan syndrome Male pattern baldness Red–green color blindness Turner syndrome Fragile X syndrome
Y-linked	Only males are affected. Mutations occur from affected fathers. Female offspring are not affected. Very rare.	Azoospermia Oligospermia Gonadal dysgenesis
Mitochondrial DNA	Also known as maternal inheritance. Only mothers can pass these disorders on to their offspring.	Leber's hereditary optic neuropathy

Major Malformations

Major malformations or birth defects are typically associated with significant physical, cognitive, or structural defects that result in some type of disability. Major birth defects include both genetic and non-genetic disorders.

Minor Malformations

Minor malformations typically have little physical or cosmetic impact and are considered harmless in and of themselves. Minor malformations often include such as low-set ears, single transverse palmar crease, telecanthus, micrognathism, macrocephaly, hypotonia and furrowed tongue. Some minor malformations are related to the presence of underlying major congenital malformations or genetic conditions; thus when they are identified, further evaluation is warranted. Patterns of major and minor malformations are found in Table 18.2.

Table 18.2

Patterns of Malformations

Type of Genetic Disorder	Description of Disorder	Examples of Disorders
Syndrome	A group of symptoms that consistently occur together or a by a set of associated symptoms	Down syndrome, Angelman Syndrome, Albinism, Congenital adrenal hyperplasia
Association	When one or more genotypes within a population co-occur with a phenotypic trait more often than would be expected by chance occurrence	Hypertriglyceridemia and atherosclerosis
Developmental Field Defect	A malformation, resulting from a dysmorphogenetic response of a developmental field	Spina bifida
Disruption	A gene knockout whereby a functional gene is replaced by an inactivated gene that is created using recombinant DNA technology. When a gene is "knocked out," the resulting mutant phenotype (observable characteristics) often reveals the gene's biological function.	
Deformations	A defect caused by an abnormal external force on the fetus during in utero development that resulted in abnormal growth, stoppage of growth, or formation of the fetal structure	Potter Sequence, Amniotic band

Parents may feel disbelief, anger, confusion, incredible sadness, blame, jealousy, heartache, emptiness, shame, a sense of unfairness, guilt, and intense grief when their newborn is diagnosed with a genetic disorder.

COMPREHENSIVE HISTORY

The genetic interview starts by taking a detailed genetic history to identify familial risk factors. During the initial visit, women should be screened for genetic risk factors and undergo a physical examination. Obtain a detailed history of the father's genetic and family history. A three-generation pedigree diagram should be constructed to outline family history. The following families warrant a referral for formal genetic counseling:

- Previous infant with genetic defect
- Family history of birth defects
- Family history of mendelian disorder
- Ethnic group risk factor
- Paternal age over 40

➡ Maternal High-Risk Conditions

The presence of certain high-risk conditions warrants further referral for genetic counseling and testing. These conditions include:

- Presence of maternal genetic defect
- Maternal age >35 at the time of birth
- History of spontaneous abortions >2
- Abnormal genetic testing results
- Maternal exposure to teratogenic risk factor
- Diabetes
- Infectious disease during pregnancy known to cause birth defects (e.g., rubella, syphilis)
- History of disorders associated with pulmonary insufficiency
- Seizures
- Maternal phenylketonuria (PKU)
- Thyroid disease

Prenatal Screening Tests

All women, regardless of age and risk factors, should be offered routine screening tests. *Screening testing* provides information to determine if a fetus is *at risk* for having a specific disorder. *Diagnostic testing* determines if the fetus is *definitely inflicted* with a specific disorder. Routine prenatal testing include:

- Maternal serum screening in the first or second trimester
- Noninvasive prenatal testing (NIPT)
- Second trimester ultrasound

If results from routine prenatal screening tests indicate an increased risk of having a baby born with a birth defect or genetic condition, offer additional diagnostic testing, including:

- Chorionic Villus Sampling
- Amniocentesis
- Percutaneous umbilical blood sampling (PUBS)

Antepartum Exposures

The antepartum is a vulnerable period for the fetus. Exposures to certain medications, environmental tetragons, or substances could put the fetus at risk for developing an abnormality. Certain antepartum events can also put the fetus at risk for a congenital defect. These risks may include:

- Medications
    - Anticonvulsants
    - Chemotherapy agents
    - Accutane
    - ACE (angiotensin-converting enzyme) inhibitors
    - High doses of vitamin A
    - Thalidomide
    - Warfarin
    - Diethylstilbestrol (DES)
    - Chloramphenicol
    - Fluoroquinolone antibiotics
    - Primaquine
    - Sulfonamides antibiotics
    - Trimethoprim
    - Ativan
    - Klonopin
    - Ibuprofen (third trimester only)

- Environmental exposures
  - Organic mercury compounds
  - Polychlorinated biphenyl (PCB)
  - Herbicides
  - Industrial solvents
  - Radiation
  - Hyperthermia

- Infectious Exposures
  - Rubella
  - Cytomegalovirus
  - Varicella
  - Herpes simplex
  - Toxoplasma
  - Syphilis
  - Listeria

- Substance exposure
  - Alcohol
  - Tobacco
  - Marijuana
  - Cocaine
  - Ecstasy
  - Amphetamines
  - Heroin
  - Opioids

Adverse Antepartum Events

- Motor vehicle accident
- Falls
- Subchorionic hemorrhage
- Umbilical cord abnormality
- Placenta previa or placenta abruptio
- Intimate partner violence or stranger assault
- Hyperthermia

Intrapartum Exposures

Intrapartum exposures occur during labor and birth and can negatively impact the fetus and increase the risk of a congenital birth injury. These may include:

- Hypoxia
- Nonreassuring fetal status
- Uterine hypersystole
- Fetal tachycardia

- Maternal fever
- Intrapartum hemorrhage or intrapartum infection
- Vacuum or forceps injury
- Delayed birth, precipitous birth, breech birth, or unattended birth
- Prolapsed umbilical cord
- Shoulder dystocia
- Preeclampsia or eclampsia
- Fetal malposition
- Macrosomia

Neonatal Factors

Certain abnormal variations that put the infant at risk for ongoing impairment may be identified or occur in the newborn period. Nurses should provide a careful assessment to identify early signs of distress, injury, or congenital abnormalities. These may include:

- Intrauterine growth restriction
- Prematurity
- Congenital anomalies

  - Hydrocephalus
  - Cleft lip/palate
  - Choanal atresia
  - Tracheoesophageal fistula
  - Diaphragmatic hernia
  - Omphalocele
  - Gastroschisis
  - Prune Belly Syndrome
  - Myelomeningocele
  - Imperforate anus
  - Clubfoot
  - Congenital hip dysplasia
  - Substance abuse or fetal alcohol syndrome

COMMONLY OCCURRING GENETIC DISORDERS

Albinism

A lack of or reduction in melanin pigment in their skin, hair, and eyes. Affected individuals have pinkish-white skin and white hair. Their eyes are usually light gray, blue, or hazel, although they may appear pink in the light. The main medical complication is poor vision and vision abnormalities.

Angelman Syndrome

A syndrome that affects the nervous system due to the absence or reduction of UBE3A. Individuals have a small head that is flat on the back, widely-spaced teeth, and eyes that look in varying directions. Severe physical and intellectual disabilities are common.

Apert Syndrome

A rare genetic condition characterized by an abnormally shaped skull and fused fingers and toes. Individuals commonly have a pointed head, broad high forehead, a sunken face, broad-set, sunken eyes, and fused fingers and toes, often with a single wide fingernail. Intellectual impairment is also common.

Charcot-Marie-Tooth Disease

A progressive neurological condition with problems of muscles of the feet, legs, arms and hands, resulting in an altered gait, weakening of leg muscles, curling of toes, hand weakness, coldness and weakness in extremities, and difficulty with fine motor skills.

Cystic Fibrosis

A genetic disease of the respiratory and digestive system. Thick mucus produces coughing, wheezing, respiratory distress, digestive problems, and thick stools.

Down Syndrome

A disorder caused by the addition of a third copy of chromosome 21. Common features include intellectual disability, low-set ears, upslanted eyes, flattened facial features, small head, ears, and mouth, short neck, and poor muscle tone.

Duchenne Muscular Dystrophy

A form of muscular degeneration caused by a mutation in the DMD gene. Dysfunction of the DMD gene leads to a lack of the protein called dystrophin, which is important for muscle strength, support, and repair. This results in difficulty walking, joint issues, and cardiac and respiratory dysfunction.

Fragile X Syndrome

Fragile X is caused by a change in a single gene, the FMR-1 gene, and results in intellectual, behavioral, and learning difficulties. It is the most commonly inherited genetic disorder and the most common cause of genetic-related autism.

Haemochromatosis

A common genetic disorder whereby too much iron is absorbed by the gut. The iron overload results in fatigue, weakness, infections, and pain. Untreated, it can lead to organ damage, infertility issues, cardiac issues, and diabetes.

Hemophilia

A genetic defect that leads to alterations in the ability of the blood to clot properly. Hemophilia A is the most common type, caused by a lack of clotting factor 8, which results from a mutation in gene F8. Hemophilia B results in lack of clotting factor 9, which results in a mutation on gene F9. Signs include frequent bruising, internal hemorrhage, heavy menses, and hemorrhage following childbirth.

Huntington's Disease

A progressive neurological disease with symptoms typically occurring in middle age, resulting in physical, cognitive, and emotional symptoms.

Klinefelter Syndrome

A genetic condition affecting males. It occurs in individuals born with an extra X chromosome. It can cause a variety of problems, including a small penis, small testes, and infertility. Individuals may have difficulty with walking, talking, learning, as well as behavioral issues.

Marfan Syndrome

A gene abnormality, characterized by a change (mutation) in the gene that affects the elasticity of both tissue that holds together muscles and joints and the connective tissue that strengthens and stabilizes joints and muscles. It generally affects the limbs but can also affect the spine, sternum, eyes, heart, and blood vessels. Individuals are often abnormally tall and thin, with longer arms and a long, thin face.

Neurofibromatosis

A genetic condition characterized by the growth of neurofibromas, a type of tumor that is usually benign or non-cancerous. The three different types originate on different genes.

Noonan Syndrome

Characterized by drooping eyelids, wide-set or sloped eyes, blue or blue-green eye color, flat-bridged nose, high-arched eyebrows, low-set ears, shortened neck, and curly, coarse hair with a low-neck hair-line. Individuals often have intellectual and behavioral problems. Symptoms typically become more pronounced with age.

Prader Willi Syndrome

A rare genetic condition caused by a genetic error at the time of con-ception and characterized by physical, behavioral, and intellectual issues. Symptoms include oversleeping, failure to thrive, poor muscle tone, weak cry, delayed milestones, and learning difficulties.

Rett Syndrome

A genetic condition of the X Chromosome, usually affecting females, affects the nervous system and results in intellectual and physical disability. Symptoms include irritability, chronic crying, and autistic-like features. They may lose their hand skills, language ability, and their ability to coordinate walking; and they may develop repetitive hand movements, such as wringing and squeezing or clapping and tapping.

Tay–Sachs Disease

A deficiency in an enzyme with the HEXA gene genetic disorder more common in Ashkenazi Jews. The disorder appears around 6 months when normal development slows, the ability to use the mus-cles ceases, and blindness occurs, resulting in childhood death by the age of 5 years old.

Thalassemia

An inherited disorder, resulting in abnormal hemoglobin. Thalassemia can be mild (often called thalassemia minor) or severe. Thalassemia causes serious problems and is called thalassemia major, Cooley's anemia, or Mediterranean anemia, depending on the genetic defect. Symptoms include lethargy, abnormal growth, shortness of breath, jaundice, deformity of facial bones, dark-colored urine, and abdominal distention.

Turner Syndrome

A disorder affecting females defined by a lack of or partial lack of the X chromosome, resulting in hearing, vision, and fertility issues. It is also known as 45, X, monosomy X, and Ullrich–Turner syndrome. Symptoms include feeding difficulties, problems with coordination, hearing or vision deficits, alterations in heart, arteries, and kidneys, slower sexual development, and puffiness in the hands and feet.

Von Willebrand Disease

A common inherited bleeding disorder, that results in difficulty controlling bleeding. The 3 types can be inherited from a parent. Symptoms include easily bruising, heavy menses, hemorrhaging after childbirth, excessive gum or nose bleeds, and bleeding into joints or muscles.

Williams Syndrome

A genetic condition present from birth characterized by developmental and learning delays, including speech delays. A small piece of chromosome 7 does not form properly after conception. Specific characteristics include a broad forehead, a small, upturned nose, a wide mouth with full lips, a small chin, and problems with the teeth. Affected children might also have weak muscles. They are prone to certain behaviors, including being overly friendly and trusting, difficulty reading social cues, tantrums, anxiety, phobias, and ADHD.

References

Davidson, M. R., Ladweig, P. L., & London, M. L. (2020). *Old's maternal newborn nursing and women's health across the lifespan* (11th ed.). Boston, MA: Pearson Education.

National Youth League Network. (2020). *Respectful disability language: Here's what's up.* Retrieved from http://www.aucd.org/docs/add/sa_summits/ Language%20Doc.pdf

19

Congenital Cardiac Defects and Critical Congenital Heart Defects

Congenital cardiac defects occur when there is an abnormality in the structure of the heart. Critical congenital heart defects are more severe in nature and typically require surgical intervention in infancy. The nurse may detect a potential defect in the first few minutes of life based on abnormal color, vital sign alternations, abnormal cardiac sounds, or difficulty with adaptation to extrauterine life.

During this part of the orientation, the nurse will be able to:

1. Compare and contrast the difference between congenital cardiac defects and critical congenital heart defects.
2. List the different types of critical congenital heart defects.
3. Differentiate the different clinical treatments and expected outcomes of the various congenital cardiac defects.
4. Outline nursing interventions for infants with cardiac defects.

Congenital cardiac defects are abnormalities in the heart's structure that occur as a result of incomplete or abnormal development in utero or as a result of a genetic defect. The incidence of congenital cardiac defects is 8 in 1,000 births. Clinical outcomes can be mild to severe in nature.

NURSING CONSIDERATIONS

- Complete physical with monitoring of heart rate and blood pressure and documentation of any cyanosis.
- Bedside pulse oximetry to determine whether critical congenital heart defect is present
- Assess for any family history of congenital cardiac disorders/disease.
- Electrocardiogram
- Echocardiogram
- Possible chest X-ray
- Possible cardiac catheterization
- Provide factual information and updates on newborn's condition.
- Referral/consultation with pediatric cardiologist
- Life-threatening cardiac defects may warrant transfer to a higher level acute care facility for intensive care services or immediate surgical intervention.
- Provide emotional support and referrals for community-based support groups/resources.
- If the infant is transferred, provide detailed referral of hospital information for parents.
- Determine whether early maternal discharge can be facilitated.

Fast Facts

Newborns with certain heart defects may warrant immediate surgical intervention and may need to be transferred to other hospital facilities that perform surgical intervention. Proper education and support for the family are imperative.

CRITICAL CONGENITAL HEART DEFECTS

Critical congenital heart defects (CCHDs) account for 30% of infant deaths related to birth defects. Infants with CCHDs often need extensive medical intervention and usually need surgical intervention within the first 12 months of life. All infants should be screened with bedside pulse oximetry 24 to 48 hours after birth (as late as possible) to check for possible CCHDs. CCHDs include:

- Coarctation of the aorta
- Double-outlet right ventricle
- D-transposition of the great arteries
- Ebstein anomaly

- Hypoplastic left heart syndrome
- Interrupted aortic arch
- Pulmonary atresia (intact septum)
- Single ventricle
- Total anomalous pulmonary venous connection
- Tetralogy of Fallot
- Tricuspid atresia
- Truncus arteriosus

Aortic Stenosis

Incidence

- 5 out of every 10,000 live births. Accounts for 5% of all congenital heart disease (Artman, Mahoney, & Tietal, 2017).

Description of Defect

- Aortic valve is stiffened with stenosis. Due to the narrowing and improper opening, the left ventricle works harder and is strained.

Clinical Treatment and Anticipated Outcome

- Mild cases do not require intervention but may warrant treatment later in life.
- Severe cases may require balloon dilation valvuloplasty via the umbilical artery. In very severe cases or when defects related to the size of the ventricles is a concern, the Ross procedure, an aortic valve replacement procedure, may be considered. The Konno procedure is sometimes considered for severe cases with severe malformations, or a Ross–Konno combination procedure may be performed.
- Prognosis is good, with children leading normal lives. A second surgery is sometimes needed later in life.

Atrial Septal Defect

Incidence

- 8 out of 10,000 births. Accounts for 8% of congenital heart disease (Artman et al., 2017).

Description of Defect

- Septum between the left atrium and the right atrium allows extra blood flow from the left atrium into the right heart and out to the lungs.

Clinical Treatment and Anticipated Outcome

- Small holes often close in the first few years of life.
- Larger septums require surgical intervention. Often, closure during a cardiac cauterization is performed. Open surgical repairs are rarely needed.
- Prognosis is excellent.

Atrioventricular Canal Defect (ACD)

Incidence

- 5% of all congenital heart disease. Present in 15% to 20% of newborns with Down syndrome.

Description of Defect

- Endocardial cushion defect; atrioventricular septal defect
- Poorly formed central area of the heart with a large hole between the atria and ventricles. Instead of two separate valves allowing flow into the heart, one large common valve, often malformed, is present instead of the tricuspid on the right and mitral valve on the left.

Clinical Treatment and Anticipated Outcome

- Common in Down syndrome
- Diuretics and angiotensin-converting enzyme (ACE) inhibitors are used, but all require surgical repair. Closures for the holes or patches are placed.
- Infants with complete ACD have surgery at 3 to 6 months and those with partial ACD can wait until 12 to 28 months.
- Survival rate is 96% and reoperation rate is 11%, with 10-year survival rates of 81% to 91% (Artman et al., 2017).

Coarctation of the Aorta

Incidence

- 5 out of 10,000 births. Accounts for 6% of congenital heart disease (Artman et al., 2017).

Description of Defect

- Narrowing of a portion of the aorta seriously decreases systemic blood flow.

Clinical Treatment and Anticipated Outcome

- Prostaglandins are often given in newborn period to stimulate heart.
- Balloon angioplasty with stent placement may be warranted.

- Good prognosis with no adverse effects is typical, although a repeat surgical procedure is sometimes needed later in life.

Hypoplastic Left Heart Syndrome

Incidence

- 1 out of every 4,344 births (Centers for Disease Control and Prevention [CDC], 2019).

Description of Defect

- Structures of the left side of the heart (the left ventricle, the mitral valve, and the aortic valve) are underdeveloped and poor systemic circulation occurs.

Clinical Treatment and Anticipated Outcome

- Diuretics may be administered and feeding tubes may be needed.
- Surgical intervention begins at 2 weeks of age with the Norwood procedure, in which a "new" aorta is constructed and connected to the right ventricle.
- A bidirectional Glenn shunt procedure is performed at 4 to 6 months to connect the pulmonary artery to the superior vena cava.
- A Fontan procedure is performed at 18 months to 3 years of age to attach the pulmonary artery to the inferior vena cava.
- Lifelong complications are common and a heart transplant is sometimes needed (CDC, 2019).

Patent Ductus Arteriosus (PDA)

Incidence

- 6 out of 10,000 births. Accounts for 7% of congenital heart disease (Artman et al., 2017).

Description of Defect

- The ductus arteriosus fails to close after birth, which results in excessive blood flow to the lungs.

Clinical Treatment and Anticipated Outcome

- Common in premature newborns.
- In preterm infants, indomethacin or ibuprofen may be given during the first 2 weeks of life to facilitate closure.
- Surgical closure is warranted during the first year if a large hole persists.
- Cardiac cauterization may be used after the first year if PDA persists and causes symptoms.
- Excellent prognosis with normal exercise tolerance expected.

Pulmonary Atresia

Incidence

- 7.1 to 8.1 per 100,000 live births. Accounts for 0.7% to 3.1% of patients with congenital heart disease (CDC, 2019).

Description of Defect

- Either absence of pulmonary valve or pulmonary valve does not open. The main blood vessel that runs between the right ventricle and the lungs might also be malformed, and the right ventricle can be abnormally small in size.

Clinical Treatment and Anticipated Outcome

- Cyanosis occurs and immediate intervention needed. Systemic-to-pulmonary artery shunt placement is performed.
- Survival rates are 65% to 82% at age 1 year and 64% to 76% at age 5 years (CDC, 2019).

Pulmonary Stenosis

Incidence

- 8 in 10,000 births. Accounts for 8% of congenital heart disease (Artman et al., 2017).

Description of Defect

- Pulmonary valve is stiffened and stenotic or does not open properly. There is potential strain on the right side of the heart because the right ventricle has to pump harder to oxygenate lungs.

Clinical Treatment and Anticipated Outcome

- If mild, pulmonary stenosis may never require any treatment.
- Prostaglandins may be given for severe narrowing. Surgical intervention via cardiac cauterization is rarely needed.
- Excellent prognosis. Follow-up surgical intervention sometimes needed later in life.

Tetralogy of Fallot

Incidence

- 5 in 10,000 births. Accounts for 5% of congenital heart disease (Artman et al., 2017).

Description of Defect

- Four defects, including a pulmonary stenosis, ventricular hypertrophy, ventricular septal defect, and an aorta that can receive blood from both the left and right ventricles instead of draining just to the left side (Eichenwald, Hansen, Martin, & Stark, 2017).

Clinical Treatment and Anticipated Outcome

- More common in DiGeorge syndrome; familial inheritance patterns
- If symptomatic, beta-blockers can be administered in newborn period. A modified Blalock–Taussig shunt may be placed.
- Open surgical repair at 6 to 12 months is common with cardiopulmonary bypass.
- Prognosis is excellent but some exercise intolerance may occur. Follow-up surgery sometimes needed.

Total Anomalous Pulmonary Venous Connection

Incidence

- 0.6 to 1.2 in 10,000 births (CDC, 2019). Accounts for 0.7% to 1.5% of congenital heart disease (CDC, 2019).

Description of Defect

- Defect in the pulmonary veins. The veins do not lead to the left atrium, but instead deliver blood to the heart by other narrowed pathways. Increased pressure pushes fluid into the lungs, decreasing oxygenated blood that reaches the body.
- Three different types: supracardiac, cardiac, and infracardiac

Clinical Treatment and Anticipated Outcome

- Respiratory distress and cyanosis may be present at birth.
- Prostaglandins are administered initially.
- If a complete obstruction is present, surgical intervention is immediate; otherwise, surgery is typically performed within 1 month.
- Prognosis is very good, although some exercise intolerance may occur.

Transposition of the Great Arteries

Incidence

- 4 in 10,000 births. Accounts for 4% of congenital heart disease (Artman et al., 2017).

Description of Defect

- Reversal of blood vessels in which the pulmonary artery and the aorta are switched. The aorta arises from the right side of the heart and receives unoxygenated blood, which then circulates through the body. The pulmonary artery arises from the left side of the heart, receives oxygenated blood, and sends it back to the lungs again.

Clinical Treatment and Anticipated Outcome

- Severe cyanosis can occur.
- Prostaglandin administration necessary during newborn period. Balloon atrial septostomy is performed via the umbilical artery. A "switch procedure" is later performed to place the arteries in the correct position.
- Prognosis is excellent.

Tricuspid Atresia

Incidence

- 1 in 10,000 births. Accounts for 0.3% to 3.7% of patients with congenital heart disease (CDC, 2019).

Description of Defect

- The tricuspid valve is replaced by a non-opening plate or membrane so the right ventricle does not receive blood normally and is often congenitally small.

Clinical Treatment and Anticipated Outcome

- Shunt procedures are typically performed during the first year of life. Digitalis and diuretics may be used if congestive heart failure occurs.
- If palliative care measures alone are used, there is a 50% fatality rate.

Truncus Arteriosus

Incidence

- 0.72 in 10,000 births. Approximately 300 cases in the United States annually (CDC, 2019).

Description of Defect

- Two separate vessels fail to form, and instead, a single common great blood vessel called the truncus arteriosus is present. A hole between the ventricles is also common. The valve leading into the truncus arteriosus may be very abnormal.

Clinical Treatment and Anticipated Outcome

- Digitalis, diuretics, and prostaglandins are commonly administered until a surgical repair can be performed. Complete primary repair is required to fix defects.
- Postoperative mortality is 10%. Survival at 10 to 20 years is 80%.

Ventricular Septal Defect

Incidence

- 3 in 1,000 births; accounts for one-third of cases of congenital heart disease (Artman et al., 2017)
- Most common congenital cardiac defect

Description of Defect

- A septum between the heart's left and right ventricles

Clinical Treatment and Anticipated Outcome

- Mild cases require no intervention. Diuretics and sometimes ACE inhibitors can be used for treatment. Large defects may require a surgical repair. Multiple small holes may require a staged repair.
- Excellent prognosis
- Close observation is warranted because irreversible lung damage can occur if not properly managed but is rare.

References

Artman, M., Mahoney, L., & Tietal, D. (2017). *Neonatal cardiology* (3rd ed.). Philadelphia, PA: McGraw-Hill Education.

Center for Disease Control and Prevention. (2019). *Data and statistics on congenital heart defects.* Retrieved from https://www.cdc.gov/ncbddd/heartdefects/data.html

Eichenwald, E. C., Hansen, A. R., Martin, C. R. & Stark, A. R. (2017). *Cloherty and Stark's manual of neonatal care* (8th ed.). Philadelphia, PA: Wolters Kluwer.

20

Physically Apparent Birth Defects

Some birth defects are apparent immediately after birth and are identified in the initial newborn examination following birth. The nurse is often the first to identify these defects and alerts the provider who has performed the birth so that the parents can be notified and educated about the condition. The nurse usually plays a vital role in helping education and support to the family in the early newborn period. Some conditions will warrant referrals to specialty providers and necessitate further testing and evaluation.

During this part of the orientation, the nurse will be able to:

1. Describe the difference between cleft lip and cleft palate.
2. List the different types of neural tube defects.
3. Define the expected outcomes of the various vascular abnormalities.
4. Outline appropriate testing strategies for infants born with sexual development abnormalities.

OROFACIAL DEFECTS

Orofacial clefts occur as an isolated defect in 70% of cases, meaning there are no other associated defects present. The incidence of cleft palate is 1 in 2,651, whereas the incidence of cleft lip with or without an associated palate is 1 in 4,437 (Centers for Disease Control and Prevention, 2020). Orofacial defects can be caused by environmental factors, genetic abnormalities, medication exposure, or nutritional deficits.

Cleft Lip Defects

- Defects occur between the fourth and seventh gestational weeks during pregnancy.
- Occur when the tissue fails to form over the lip
- Can be a small slit or large opening
- Often unilateral but can occur in the middle of the lip (rare)

Cleft Palate Defects

- Defects occur between sixth and ninth gestational weeks during pregnancy.
- Occur when the tissue that makes up the roof of the mouth does not join correctly
- Can include the front and back portion or a small section of the palate

Complications Related to Cleft Lip and Cleft Palate

- Feeding difficulties
- Speech delays/alterations
- Dental problems
- Ear infections
- Hearing loss

Nursing Considerations

- Assess for the presence of other birth defects.
- Parents need factual information about the defects.
- Parents need emotional support and opportunities to grieve.
- Consultation with a surgeon about a plan of care should be scheduled early.
- Because breathing, hearing, speech, and language can be affected, referrals to appropriate specialists are warranted.
- Feeding consultation is warranted for feeding issues.
- Lactation consultation is warranted as breastfeeding may difficult (sometimes not possible).
- Specialized bottles should be provided to aid in feeding.
- Close observation for adequate fluid intake and weight gain are important as feeding difficulties are common.
- Hearing screening is especially important in this population.

- Surgical consultation.
- Prompt surgery may be warranted if breathing or other severe complications are present.
- Surgical intervention is warranted by 12 months for infants with cleft lip and 18 months for infants with cleft palate.

NEURAL TUBE DEFECTS (NTDS)

NTDs occur during the 18 to 23 gestational day period and can result in primary NTDs or secondary NTDs. The range of adverse complications is directly correlated to the type of degree of the defects. The incidence if 1;2,000 with multiple etiologies including folate deficiency, genetic variables, use of certain medications (anti-convulsant, ant-malarial drugs), maternal diabetes, irradiation in early pregnancy, and maternal hyperthermia (Eichenwald, Hansen, Martin, & Stark, 2017). Table 20.1 outlines the different types of NTDs.

Adverse Effects and Complications

Adverse effects vary significantly based on the type of defect that is present.
- Infection from leaking open placode
- Hydrocephalus from increased intracranial pressure
- Need for shunt placement
- Failure to thrive
- Feeding difficulties
- Seizures
- Fluid and electrolyte imbalances from leaking membrane

Table 20.1

Primary and Secondary Neural Tube Defects	
Primary NTDs	**Secondary NTDs**
Myelomeningocele	Meningocele
Encephalocele	Lipomeningocele
Anencephaly	Filum lipoma
	Sacral agenesis/degenesis
	Diastematomyelia
	Myelocyctocele

- Incomplete bladder emptying
- Neurogenic bladder
- Bladder and bowel incontinence
- Frequent urinary tract infections
- Sensory impairment
- Respiratory complications
- Congenital hip dysplasia
- Foot deformities
- Walking ability deteriorates with increased age
- Back pain
- Scoliosis
- Chronic leg pain; muscle spasms
- Paralysis
- Orthopedic abnormalities
- Cardiac Malformations
- Spinal defects
- Arnold Chiari II malformations
- Seizures
- Visual impairment
- Learning disabilities
- Attention deficit disorder
- Impaired perceptual motor skills
- Impaired memory and organizational skills
- Difficulties with numeric reasoning
- Precocious puberty
- Sexual dysfunction
- Latex allergy

Nursing Considerations

- Obtain a detailed family and pregnancy history.
- Comprehensive physical assessment
- Position in a prone position with legs slightly flexed and bent.
- Cover the lesion with moistened gauze.
- Record head circumference daily.
- Observe for seizures.
- Obtain necessary consultations.

    - Surgery
    - Neurology
    - Genetics
    - Urology
    - Orthopedics
    - Physical therapy
    - Social work

- Pastoral services
- Speech therapy (for feeding difficulties)

- Ongoing assessment for meningitis and infection

  - Administer intravenous antibiotics

- MRI or CT
- Hearing screen
- Vision assessment
- Observe for feeding difficulties
- Daily weights
- Urinary cultures and urinalysis
- Renal ultrasound
- Postvoid residual monitoring
- Radiographic studies of spine, lower limbs, and hips
- Coordination of interdisciplinary care services
- Referral for home care services
- Referral to specialty clinic or developmental pediatrician

Fast Facts

Parents with infants with birth defects should be provided with resources including psychological support, peer support groups, online professional organization for medical information, and referrals for counseling as needed.

ORTHOPEDIC CONDITIONS

Congenital orthopedic impairments occur in approximately 1% of all live births. There are a variety of orthopedic conditions. Treatment depends on the type of condition and the extent of impairment it may cause.

Congenital Muscular Torticollis (CMT)

CMT is characterized by limited head movement, limited motions of the neck, asymmetrical face and skull, and a tilted position of the head. The condition can be due to intrauterine position or over-stretching of the head and neck during the birth. Treatment includes positioning and passive stretching. A helmet is sometimes indicated with severe head asymmetry.

Polydactyly

Polydactyly is often the result of an autosomal dominant inheritance, although inherited syndromes may also be an etiological factor and indicate a more serious underlying origin. Digits with no bone or cartilage are typically tied off and allowed to fall off secondary to necrosis. Digits on the thumb side of medial border of the foot, along with those that contain cartilage or bone, warrant surgical consultation for removal within the first 6 to 12 months after birth.

Congenital and Infantile Scoliosis

Congenital scoliosis occurs when there is an abnormality in the formation of the vertebra or a segment of the vertebra. Infantile scoliosis differs in that there is a curvature with no vertebral anomaly. It typically improves without treatment. Congenital scoliosis often requires body casting. Surgical intervention is warranted if respiratory compromise exists. Ultrasound determines if there are renal or organ abnormalities.

Congenital Hip Locations (CHLs)

CHLs can be identified at birth and are a result of one of three different anatomical variations.

Classic developmental hip dysplasia is a unilateral hip dysplasia that is characterized by a positive Ortolani sign, a symmetrical pelvis, and the presence of a hip dislocation that is present on flexion and extension, but relocates when the femur is abducted.

Teratologic hip dislocation occurs as a result of early failure of the femoral head to relocate on flexion and extension.

Congenital abduction contracture occurs later in pregnancy and results in a unilateral dislocation that causes a pelvis irregularity.

Nursing Considerations

- Classic Developmental Hip Dislocation

    - Most commonly unilateral but can be bilateral
    - More common in females
    - Often resolves by 5 days of life
    - Positioning with splint to facilitate hip flexion and abduction is warranted after 5 days
    - Pavlik Harness may be used
    - Ultrasound assessment of ongoing progress is warranted.

- Teratologic Dislocation

  - Ortolani sign is not present
  - May be unilateral or bilateral
  - Limited abduction at birth suggests diagnosis.
  - Open surgical reduction
  - Exercise is recommended, but a Pavlik Harness is not beneficial.

- Congenital Abduction Contracture

  - Development of a short leg and asymmetrical gluteal folds occur by 6 weeks.
  - Hip subluxate may occur.
  - Initial treatment with Pavlik Harness is appropriate up until 8 months of age.

Genu Recurvatum

Genu recurvatum, or hyperextension of the knee, should be differentiated from a true knee dislocation or subluxation.

Nursing Considerations

- Radiographic studies can differentiate between genu recurvatum and true knee dislocation or subluxation.
- Congenital fibrosis of the quadriceps is a common co-morbidity requiring open reduction.
- It is treated with repeated casting with progressive flexion of the knee.
- Hyperextended and subluxated knees are treated with manipulation and splinting.
- Fixed dislocation requires open reduction.

Metartarsus Adductus

- Metatarsals rest in an adducted position.
- Occurs due to positional deformities from utero positioning
- Self-limiting without treatment
- Structural metatarsal adductus is a fixed state with no passive adduction.

  - Treated with manipulation and immobilization

Calcaneovalgus Deformities

- In utero positioning that results in holding an ankle dorsiflexed and in abducted position
- Treatment with exercise or short leg cast
- Serial casting is sometimes warranted.

Congenital Clubfoot

- Foot is equinus, cavus, and varus position with forefoot abduction
- Passive manipulation is not possible
- Occurs more frequently in firstborn children, oligohydramnios, or as part of a syndrome, such as spina bifida
- Weekly casting is warranted, with treatment beginning as soon as possible after birth.
- Bracing is warranted until age 4.
- Physical therapy and splitting

COMPARTMENT SYNDROME OF THE NEWBORN

Compartment syndrome is a rare and serious condition with an unknown etiology resulting in an edematous arm with skin lesions. Prompt surgical intervention can help prevent scarring, disability, nerve injury, and loss or partial loss of the affected limb.

VASCULAR ABNORMALITIES

Vascular abnormalities may include vascular tumors or vascular malformations.

Infantile Hemangioma

- Red or bluish tumor appears by 2 weeks of age involving the superficial dermis.

Nursing Considerations

- Advise parents of increasing size and rapid growth during first 9 months with full size typically reached by 9 months. Regression begins at 12 months and disappearance by 4 years of age.
- Monitor for presence of five or more hemangiomas, which can indicate liver involvement. If liver involvement suspected, TSH monitoring is warranted. If treatment is warranted, order topical, intralesional, or systemic pharmacotherapy.

Congenital Hemangioma

- Red violaceous lesions with a pale halo exterior portion. Rapidly involuting congenital hemangioma (RICH) and noninvoluting congenital hemangioma (NICH)

Nursing Considerations

- Advise parents RICH typically resolves by 7 to 14 months but may persist longer. If rapid blood flow present, observe for signs and symptoms of CHF. NICH remains present and may require resection for cosmetic issues.

Kaposiform Hemangioendothelioma

- Rare nonmetastasizing vascular neoplasm with a red, purplish, flat edematous appearance

Nursing Considerations

- Assess CBC and observe for bleeding and petechiae as Kasabach-Merritt exists in up to 70% of affected infants. Observe for active bleeding. Platelet transfusions are often unsuccessful and are only ordered with active bleeding or if surgery is planned.
- Administer vincristine. Advise parents resolution typically occurs by 2 years of age but residual pain and stiffness are common.

Capillary Malformation (Port Wine Stain)

Pink-purplish skin discoloration

Nursing Considerations

- Reassure parents it does not have adverse effects but may darken, and infant have soft tissue and bone enlargement under the mark. Discuss the use of pulse dye laser, which can be administered during infancy to lighten the stain.

Lymphatic Malformation

- Lesions that are characterized by their channels

Nursing Considerations

- Observe for signs of infection or bleeding. Sclerotherapy can treat smaller lesions and needle aspiration for larger ones. Obtain an MRI for deep lesions.

Venous Malformations

- Bluish soft compressible lesions

Nursing Considerations

- Obtain MRI for large, deep lesions; most require no diagnostic work-up. Sclerotherapy is the treatment of choice after 12 months of age. The Risk of thromboembolism is low, but aspirin therapy can be used for pain and prevention of phlebothrombosis.

Arteriovenous Malformation

■ Pink-red cutaneous pulsating lesion with warmth that results in shunting from the arterial to venous circulation

Nursing Considerations

■ Obtain a doppler examination and MRI or angiogram if needed. Ongoing observation is required; embolization is performed. Resection may be done but is not the first line of therapy.

SEXUAL DEVELOPMENT ABNORMALITIES

Disorders of sexual development (DOD) is a term used to describe a broad group abnormal development that may have etiologies related to genetics, gonad malformation, or anatomical variations in sex organs that make gender identity difficult to determine (Michigan Medicine, 2020).

Types of DOD

■ Ambiguous genitalia
■ Cryptorchidism (penis with nonpalpable testes)
■ Unilateral cryptorchidism with hypospadias
■ Severe penoscrotal, scrotal, or perineal hypospadias
■ Female appearance with enlarged clitoris (and/or inguinal hernia and palpable gonads)
■ Asymmetrical female characteristics including size, pigmentation, or rogation of labia folds
■ External genitalia does not match prenatal karyotype

MIXED GONADAL DSYGENESIS

Mixed gonadal dysgenesis (MGD) is associated with an abnormal karyotype that results in mixed genitalia on one side of the body and a streak or abnormal gonad on the other (Michigan Medicine, 2020).

Types of MGD

■ Mosaic karyotypes (45X/46XY)
■ Swyer Syndrome (complete gonadal dysgenesis; 46 XY)

- Testicular DSD (46XX)
- Ovotesticular DSD (Mosaic 46 XX with 10% 46 XY)
- CAH

Adverse Effects

- Significant family distress
- Congenital adrenal hyperplasia
- Genetic defects
- Mismatch between external and internal sex anatomy

Nursing Considerations for Infants With MGD

- Obtain a comprehensive family history.
- An endocrinology consult is warranted as soon as possible.
- Comprehensive expert genital assessment is obtained.
- Provide education and support for parents.
- Obtain diagnostic testing.

  - Chromosomal analysis
  - Pelvic ultrasound
  - VCUG
  - Hormonal testing

- Wait to assign sex until laboratory and diagnostic testing is obtained.
- Encourage parents not to assign name or sex until a recommendation for future sex assignment has been determined.
- The timing of surgical interventions is controversial.
- Encourage parents to seek a specialist in the area of DOD as early as possible.

References

Centers for Disease Control and Prevention. (2020). *Facts about cleft lip and cleft palate.* Retrieved from https://www.cdc.gov/ncbddd/birthdefects/cleftlip.html

Eichenwald, E. C., Hansen, A. R., Martin, C. R., & Stark, A. R. (2017). *Cloherty and Stark's manual of neonatal care* (8th ed.). Philadelphia, PA: Wolters Kluwer.

Michigan Medicine. (2020). *Disorders of sexual development.* Retrieved from https://www.med.umich.edu/yourchild/topics/dsd.htm

21

Underlying Birth Defects

Underlying birth defects include disorders that are not readily apparent at the time of birth via physical examination. Some conditions will not be known until the newborn is born. In modern obstetrics, some of these conditions are identified in utero by ultrasound. In these cases, careful follow-up in the neonatal period is warranted. In cases without a known diagnosis, specialty referrals and consultations are often warranted.

During this part of the orientation, the nurse will be able to:

1. Identify the different types of inborn errors of metabolism.
2. List common gastrointestinal abnormalities.
3. Differentiate between kidney and liver abnormalities.
4. Compare and contrast the different hematological conditions that can present in the newborn period.
5. Discuss the different thyroid disorders that can affect the newborn.

INBORN ERRORS OF METABOLISM

Individual inborn errors of metabolism (IEMs) are relatively rare but life-threatening. They result from single-gene defects. IEM disorders can involve toxic accumulation or may be related to energy production/utilization disorders. Individual IEMs are rare, although collectively, they occur in 1 in 4,000 births. The most common IEMs are listed in Table 21.1.

Table 21.1

Inborn Errors of Metabolism

Type of IEM	Incidence	Clinical Symptomology	Inheritance Pattern
Phenylketonuria	1:15,000	Intellectual disability, microcephaly	Autosomal recessive
Maple syrup urine disease	1:150,000	Acute encephalopathy, metabolic acidosis, intellectual disability	Autosomal recessive
Galactosemia	1:40,000	Hepatocellular dysfunction, cataracts	Autosomal recessive
Glycogen storage disease, type Ia (von Gierke's disease)	1:100,000	Hypoglycemia, lactic acidosis, ketosis	Autosomal recessive
Medium-chain acyl-CoA dehydrogenase deficiency	1:15,000	Nonketotic hypoglycemia, acute encephalopathy, coma, sudden infant death syndrome	Autosomal recessive
Pyruvate dehydrogenase deficiency	1:200,000	Hypotonia, psychomotor retardation, failure to thrive, seizures, lactic acidosis	X-linked
Gaucher's disease	1:60,000 (increased to 1:1,900 in Ashkenazi Jews)	Coarse facial features, hepatosplenomegaly	Autosomal recessive
Fabry's disease	1:80,000–1:117,000	Acroparesthesias, angiokeratomas, hypohidrosis, corneal opacities, renal insufficiency	X-linked
Hurler's syndrome	1:100,000	Coarse facial features, hepatosplenomegaly	Autosomal recessive

(continued)

Table 21.1

Inborn Errors of Metabolism (*continued*)

Type of IEM	Incidence	Clinical Symptomology	Inheritance Pattern
Methylmalonica ciduria	1:20,000	Acute encephalopathy, metabolic acidosis, hyperammonemia	Autosomal recessive
Propionic aciduria	1:50,000	Metabolic acidosis, hyperammonemia	Autosomal recessive
Zellweger syndrome	1:50,000	Hypotonia, seizures, liver dysfunction	Autosomal recessive
Ornithine transcarbamylase deficiency	1:70,000	Acute encephalopathy	X-linked

Toxic Accumulation Defects

- Disorders of protein metabolism (amino acidopathies, organic acidopathies, urea cycle defects)
- Disorders of carbohydrate intolerance
- Lysosomal storage disorders

Energy Production and Utilization Defects

- Fatty acid oxidation defects
- Disorders of carbohydrate utilization or production (glycogen storage disorders; disorders of gluconeogenesis and glycogenolysis)
- Mitochondrial disorders
- Peroxisomal disorders

Adverse Effects and Complications

- Acute sepsis with no risk factors (occurs in 20% of affected newborns)
- Temperature instability
- Rapid deterioration after initial normal newborn course
- Neurological changes

    - Severe onset of ataxia
    - Seizures
    - Irregular movements

- Posturing
- Abnormal tone
- Altered/changes in level of consciousness

- Hepatoencephalopathy
- Organomegaly
- Poor perfusion
- Tachypnea
- Bradycardia
- Apnea
- Acute organ dysfunction
- Multisystem organ failure
- Feeding/gastrointestinal changes

  - Poor feeding
  - Vomiting
  - Failure to thrive
  - Lethargy

- Developmental delays
- Failure to reach developmental milestones/loss of milestones
- Skeletal deformities

  - Dysmorphic features
  - Skeletal abnormalities

- Cardiopulmonary compromise
- Coma
- Unexplained newborn/infant death

Nursing Considerations for the Care of Newborns With IEM

- Obtain an extensive family history (including a family history of unexplained newborn/infant death).
- Ensure tandem mass spectrometry testing is performed as late as possible prior to discharge.
- The Initial physical exam may be normal, but alterations can begin occurring as early as 24 hours after birth, with rapid deterioration common.
- Immediately transfer to a tertiary care facility.
- If IEMs are suspected, comprehensive laboratory testing includes complete blood count; serum electrolytes; bicarbonate; blood gases; blood urea nitrogen; creatinine levels; bilirubin level; transaminase levels; prothrombin time; activated partial thromboplastin time; blood glucose; lactate dehydrogenase; aldolase; creatinine kinase; and urinary testing, including pH, ketones, and urine myoglobin levels.

- Imaging studies may include electrocardiogram, radiography, computed tomography, magnetic resonance imaging, ultrasonography, and/or echocardiogram.
- Obtain enzyme assay or DNA analysis.
- If laboratory findings are abnormal, prompt consultation with an IEM specialist is warranted.
- Obtain guidelines and algorithms from the American College of Medical Genetics.
- If newborn death occurs, diagnostic testing should be performed to determine risk factors for future pregnancies and screening for siblings who could be asymptomatic.
- Emergency treatment includes immediate NPO (nothing orally) status, intravenous D10 to stabilize blood sugar levels, correction of metabolic acidosis if present, elimination of toxic metabolites, and administration of cofactors specific for the treatment of IEM.
- Some IEMs will require specific replacement enzymes.
- Specialized formulas are required and individualized based on the specific type of IEM.
- Referrals for psychological counseling and community-based support are warranted.
- Organ transplants, enzyme therapy, and gene therapy required as needed
- Extensive parent education is imperative.
- Lifelong management required
- Dietary strategies typically include protein restriction and avoidance of fasting.
- Stressors, including dietary changes, trauma, or surgery, can worsen symptoms.

Fast Facts

Every state is required by law to screen for at least 29 IEMs. Some states screen for over 50 IEMs. Screening thresholds are intentionally set low to avoid false negatives, so false positives can occur.

GASTROINTESTINAL ABNORMALITIES

Gastrointestinal obstruction can be congenital, acquired, or functional. Intervention is based on identifying the type of obstruction present (Eichenwald, Hansen, Martin, & Stark, 2017). Table 21.2 lists the different types of obstructions that occur.

Table 21.2

Types of Gastrointestinal Obstruction

Congenital	Acquired	Functional
Intrinsic atresias (duodenal)	Malrotation of the volvulus	Immature bowel mobility
Intrinsic stenosis	Strictures related to NEC	Defective bowel wall innervation
Meconium ileus		
Small left colon syndrome	Peritoneal adhesions	Paralytic ileus
Lumen bowel cysts	Incarcerated inguinal hernia	Meconium ileus (associated with cystic fibrosis)
Imperforate anus	Hypertrophic pyloric stenosis	Meconium plug
Congenial peritoneal bands	Mesenteric thrombosis	Mucous plug
Annular pancreas	Intussusception	Abnormal intestinal concretions
Intestinal duplications	Gastroschisis	
Aberrant vessels		
Hydrometrocolpos		
Obstructing bands		

Adverse Effects and Complications

- Genetic defects
- Cardiovascular defects
- Gastrointestinal malformations
- Cystic fibrosis
- Feeding issues
- Shock
- Sepsis

Nursing Considerations for Infants With Gastrointestinal Abnormalities

- Perform a comprehensive assessment.
- Observe for profuse vomiting.
- Observe for bilious emesis.
- Place nasogastric sump tube.
- Monitor bilirubin levels.
- Administer phototherapy as indicated.
- Obtain testing for co-existing anomalies or disorders.

- Test for cystic fibrosis.
- Perform an X-ray the stomach.
- Perform an abdominal ultrasound.
- Obtain an UGI series

- Administer intravenous antibiotics.
- Administer contrast enemas.
- Maintain adequate hydration prior to contrast studies.
- Initiate treatment protocol for Meconium/mucous plugs.

- Insert glycerin suppositories
- Warm and administer half saline enemas.
- Provide rectal stimulation
- Administer a contrast enema
- Obtain a surgical consultation
- Prepare for immediate surgery for certain conditions.

KIDNEY ABNORMALITIES

Kidney abnormalities can occur as a result of genetic variations or functional developmental issues. Any newborn with a suspected genetic etiology should undergo a clinical kidney assessment to determine if there is an alteration in kidney anatomy or function. Abdominal, renal, genital, and gastrointestinal masses may also alter renal functioning and warrant a comprehensive renal assessment. Congenital anomalies of kidney and urinary tract (CAKUT) is a broad term used to describe different disorders associated with the kidneys or urinary tract. The incidence of CAKUT is 1 in 100 to 1 in 500 (Eichenwald et al., 2017).

Hydronephrosis

Incidence

- 2 to 2.5% with a higher incidence in boys

Nursing Considerations

- Obtain renal ultrasound after birth if bilateral is suspected or was identified prenatally.
- Follow-up between 2 to 4 by 4 weeks of age is required.
- In male infants:

- Assess for abdominal mass; obtain a VCUG to determine etiology; administer antibiotics until etiology established and posterior urethral valves (PUV) is ruled out. If PUV present, a long-term antibiotic regimen is recommended.

Multicyclic Dysplastic Kidney (Polycystic Kidney Disease)

Incidence

- 1 in 3,640 births

Nursing Considerations

- Obtain prenatal and family history.
- Assess for abdominal mass and distention. Assessment via ultrasound is warranted.
- Obtain liver, bile duct, and genetic studies
- Assess for renal insufficiency.
- Surgical removal is sometimes performed due to infection or respiratory compromise related to abdominal compression.
- Long-term consultation with ongoing assessment is recommended throughout life. Kidney transplant is sometimes indicated in later life.

Acute Kidney Injury (AKI), Prerenal Azotemia, Intrinsic AKI (Rare in Newborns), Postrenal AKI

Incidence

- 8% of infants admitted to NICU

Nursing Considerations

- Assess for prenatal risk factors and nephrotoxic medication use.
- Monitor urinary output via an indwelling catheter.
- Evaluate for signs of intravascular depletion; oliguria is the initial symptom and warrants close observation of input and output.
- Obtain serum creatinine levels.
- Assess for edema; conduct fluid challenge test to determine if intravascular depletion is occurring.
- Obtain renal ultrasound and lab studies including urine sodium, plasma creatinine, and fractured excretion of sodium (FENa).
- Administer intravenous albumin if ordered.
- Assess and manage blood pressure variations.
- Initiate low potassium intake and formula.
- Calcium administration, sodium bicarbonate, insulin, and glucose will temporarily lower potassium levels and may be ordered.
- Manage fluid and provide nutritional assessment. Dialysis may be needed.

Anomalies of the Kidneys: Renal Agenesis, Renal Hypoplasia, Renal Dysplasia, Horseshoe Kidney, Kidney Malposition, Polycystic Kidney Disease

Incidence

- 1 in 100 to 1 in 500 (CAKUT)

Nursing Considerations

- Obtain family and pregnancy history.
- Assess for genetic etiologies through genetic testing.
- Comprehensive physical assessment may reveal an inability to palpate the kidney.
- Assess for dysmorphic features.
- Observe for signs of urinary tract infection, abdominal distention, edema, poor feeding, and poor growth.
- Monitor intake and output.
- Obtain urinalysis and urine culture, kidney function testing, and CBC.
- Antibiotic therapy is often necessary.
- Facilitate diagnostic testing: CT or MRI of the kidneys and urinary tract, ultrasound, renal scan, and voiding cystourethrogram (VCUG).
- Renal biopsy is sometimes warranted.

Anomalies of the Ureters: Ureteropelvic Junction Obstruction, Ureterovesical Junction Obstruction or Ureterocele, Vesicoureteral Reflux

Incidence

- 1 in 100 to 1 in 500 (CAKUT)

Nursing Considerations

- Obtain a family history and perform a comprehensive physical exam, monitoring intake and output, inability to void, abdominal distention, ascites, edema, and poor feeding.
- Antibiotics may be warranted to prevent backflow.
- Lab studies include urinalysis, urine culture, and kidney function testing.
- Obtain diagnostic testing: CT or MRI of the kidneys and urinary tract, ultrasound, renal scan, and VCUG.
- A surgical consult may be indicated.

Anomalies of the Urethra

Incidence

- 1 in 100 to 1 in 500 (CAKUT)

Nursing Considerations

- Obtain familial history of CAKUT or other congenital anomalies.
- Perform a comprehensive physical exam, monitoring intake and output, inability to void, abdominal distention, ascites, suprapubic mass, edema, and poor feeding.
- Surgical intervention may be warranted if a complete blockage is present.
- Antibiotics often are used due to frequent infections.

Tubular Disorders: Fanconi Syndrome: Renal Tubular Acidosis: Nephrocalcinosis

Incidence

- Common in premature infants

Nursing Considerations

- Obtain history and assess for sickle cell disease and autoimmune disorders like lupus and Sjogren syndrome.
- Observe for symptoms including respiratory distress, tachypnea, tachycardia, vomiting, failure to thrive, hematuria, and polyuria.
- Assess for the presence of abnormal potassium calcium levels, glucose, bicarbonate, phosphate, amino acids, and vitamin D abnormalities.
- Observe for liver abnormalities, failure to thrive, growth restriction, and metabolic acidosis.
- Assess all medication administered during the neonatal period.
- Facilitate alkali treatment as ordered. Treatment of the underlying cause is the mainstay of treatment.

THYROID DISORDERS

Thyroid disorders in neonates are almost exclusively limited to newborns of women with Grave's disease, with an incidence of 1% to 2%. The most common thyroid conditions affecting the newborn is neonatal goiter and congenital hypothyroidism.

Neonatal Goiter

- Often diagnosed during pregnancy
- Most common cause is moderate to severe Grave's disease or low dosing of medication during pregnancy
- Other causes include thyroid-stimulating hormone (TSH), receptor-stimulating antibodies, thyroid hormonogenesis disorders, excessive iodine ingestion, and maternal iodine deficiency

Adverse Effects and Complications

- Genetic defects
- Sensorineural hearing loss
- Hyperthyroidism
- Hypothyroidism
- Respiratory compromise
- Swallowing difficulties

Nursing Considerations

- Assess the thyroid size and presence of nodules.
- Obtain thyroid panel as thyroid functioning can be normal, hypoactive, or hyperactive.
- Assess if respiratory distress is present due to pressure on airway.
- Surgical consult with intervention warranted if respiratory impairment is present.
- Genetic consultation is indicated since 15% occur due to genetic mutations.
- Conduct hearing screening since some genetic variations can result in hearing loss.
- Treatment during pregnancy or after delivery with L-thyroxine reduces goiter size.

Fast Facts

Carefully assess the thyroid gland and be alert to the size of a thyroid goiter as gross enlargement can put pressure on the airway and result in respiratory depression or respiratory arrest.

Hypothyroidism

Inadequate thyroid production may occur due to an anatomical defect, inborn error of thyroid metabolism, or an iodine deficiency. The disorder occurs in 1 in 1,500 births.

Adverse Effects

- Developmental and language delays; learning and intellectual disability
- Macroglossia
- Goiter
- Anemia
- Myxedema
- Impaired linear bone growth
- Muscle spasticity
- Gait abnormalities
- Mutism
- Autism
- Visuospatial difficulties
- Fine motor function alterations
- Memory deficits
- Attention issues

Nursing Considerations

- Observe for coarse facial features, large fontanelles, umbilical hernia, and pallor.
- Assess for thyroid goiter.
- Obtain serum thyroid hormone (total or free T4) and elevated levels of TSH.
- Assess for the presence of maternal and neonatal antithyroid antibodies.
- Evaluate for thyroid-binding globulin (TBG) deficiency.
- Obtain a thyroid scan or an ultrasound scan.
- Obtain a lateral x-ray of the knee to assess for distal femoral epiphysis.
- Provide thyroid replacement hormone therapy.

Reference

Eichenwald, E. C., Hansen, A. R., Martin, C. R., & Stark, A. R. (2017). *Cloherty and Stark's manual of neonatal care* (8th ed.). Philadelphia, PA: Wolters Kluwer.

VII

The NICU

22

Introduction to the Neonatal Intensive Care Unit (NICU)

The care of high-risk newborns and their families occurs most commonly in the neonatal intensive care unit. Family-centered developmentally supportive care models embrace care of the newborn and focus on the developmental needs along with the care required for the entire family unit. Infants in the NICU often face invasive procedures that require pain-relieving strategies to keep them comfortable. The nurse plays an important role in the preparation of the infant and the education of parents when invasive procedures are needed. Some critically ill infants often warrant interventions that will involve neonatal surgery. The neonate represents multiple challenges when undergoing surgical intervention, including the use of anesthesia when the newborn is not stable. Many of these newborns will need to be transferred to facilities that can meet their unique care needs.

During this part of the orientation, the nurse will be able to:

1. Describe the concept of family-centered developmentally supportive care.
2. Identify interventions to reduce pain for the newborn undergoing invasive procedures.
3. List common neonatal procedures performed in the NICU.
4. Discuss issues that occur related to newborn transport.
5. Outline common concerns related to the use of anesthesia for surgical interventions in the newborn period.

FAMILY-CENTERED DEVELOPMENTALLY SUPPORTIVE CARE

Family-centered developmentally supportive care (FCDSC) is a holistic interdisciplinary approach that recognizes the neonate as a human being in his/her own right, and the newborn and family as a single entity. This philosophical approach improves family and neonatal outcomes through comprehensive care partnerships between professional staff and families while maintaining a family's diversity and dignity, and providing respect. In this model of care, the current needs of the infant and the family guide the staff to provide developmentally-supported care, which includes facilitating kangaroo care, skin-to-skin contact, early breastfeeding and pumping, rooming-in, and allowing parents to provide hands-on care of the infant, including those with fragile medical needs.

FCDSC is hallmarked by the following characteristics (Ramazani, Shirazi, Sarvestani, & Moiattani, 2014; Westrup, 2015):

- Family assessment to determine their needs
- Caretaking of the family by providing for their needs
- Equal family participation in decision-making for neonatal care
- Professional and family collaboration with care planning, discharge planning, and long-term needs
- Respect of family's differences and preferences for care practices and decisions
- Empowerment through being active team members and having decision-making input in neonatal care.

ENVIRONMENTAL, FACILITY & EDUCATIONAL FACTORS

Environmental factors, facility resources, and educational resources in the NICU can provide the family with comforts and conveniences that will promote their comfort, reduce anxiety, provide resources that allow them to spend time with their newborn to facilitate attachment, increase physical and emotional comfort, provide opportunities to promote rest and healing, and gain empowerment through knowledge and education. These resources may include:

- Rooming-in facilities
- Sleep rooms for parents and caregivers
- Sleep chairs, comfortable rockers, breastfeeding stools, breastfeeding cushions
- Kitchen area for food storage or preparation
- Donated meals, snacks, and drinks
- Breast pumping room

- Written resources including books, pamphlets, brochures (in native language)
- Educational visual technology programming channels for education
- Volunteers to rock neonates and provide kangaroo care in parent's absence
- Support groups
- PMAD (postpartum mood and anxiety disorder) screenings for parents
- Sibling visitation policies to promote family attachment
- Chaplain or spiritual resources
- Peer support programs and resources
- Nurse-led educational sessions
- Car seat safety education

NEONATAL TRANSPORT

Neonatal transport is sometimes warranted if an infant requires care or surgical intervention not available at the delivering facility. U.S. hospitals have three levels of nursery units, although some regions will designate hospitals based on a four-tier division:

- Well baby (Level I NICU)

  - Newborns born after 35 weeks
  - Newborns in stable condition

- Special care nursery (Level II NICU)

  - Newborns born after 32 weeks
  - Provides monitoring after birth
  - Intravenous fluids and medications
  - Temperature stability
  - Premature infants
  - Jaundice

- Level III NICU

  - Care for any gestational age
  - Provides respiratory support
  - Intravenous fluids and medications
  - Tube feedings

- Level IV NICU

  - Care of threshold-of-viability newborns
  - Intensive respiratory support
  - Neonatal surgery

Perinatal Regionalization System

Perinatal regionalization is a system designating where infants are born or are transferred after birth based on the amount of care they need. In regionalized systems, very ill or very small infants are placed in facilities that provide the highest level of care with high-level technology and specialized health providers on site. Whenever possible, mothers are sent to the most appropriate medical facility to care for the needs of the newborn prior to delivery; however, not all pregnant women can be safely transferred prior to birth and neonatal transfer may be needed.

Essential Skills of the Neonatal Transport Team

Neonates may need immediate transfer upon delivery to obtain the most appropriate care. Transport can include ground, helicopter, or airplane transport options. During transport, stabilization, therapeutic hypothermia, ventilation, continuous monitoring, and drug administration may be needed. Nurses on neonatal transport teams need to provide precise critical thinking skills and possess extensive clinical expertise.

PREPARATION FOR INVASIVE PROCEDURES

Preparation for procedures in the NICU, whenever possible, should begin with providing the parents with a comprehensive overview of the procedure being performed, the risks and benefits of the procedure, potential alternatives, and obtaining informed consent. The neonate should be monitored by a secondary care provider throughout the procedure and pain control interventions should be administered. A time-out, safety check or pauses, and checklist should be used to reduce medical errors.

Neonatal Pain Control

Pain control in neonates can be managed through non-pharmacological interventions such as sucking sweet-tasting water, breastfeeding, and nonnutritive sucking. Pharmacological interventions should be considered for procedures longer than 5 minutes or associated with higher levels of discomfort and pain. These may include topical anesthetics, analgesics, opioid analgesia, and sedatives. The type of pharmacological use is determined by the gestational age, type of procedure, and risk factors present (Eichenwald, Hansen, Martin, & Stark, 2017).

Fast Facts

The nurse plays a valuable role in advocating for nonpharmacological pain relief measures. Rubbing the newborn's hand or providing glucose water and talking to the newborn in a low soothing voice can provide comfort during painful procedures.

COMMON NEONATAL PROCEDURES

The procedures listed below utilize nonpharmacological pain interventions. Some procedures may require pharmacological medications due to the heightened pain level associated with certain procedures.

Phlebotomy

- Capillary blood is drawn from the warmed lateral side of the sole of the foot using a spring-loaded lancet after cleaning.
- Venous blood is most easily obtained from the antecubital or saphenous veins after careful cleaning.
- Arterial blood is typically drawn from the radial artery or posterior tibial artery with a 25 G needle using transillumination.
- Catheter blood samples are obtained from the umbilical or radial artery catheter using a needless system after careful cleaning. Withdrawing infusate is required to obtain accurate values.

Bladder Catheterization

- Cleaning of the urethra and suprapubic area
- Insertion of a 3 to 5 French catheter under sterile technique.

Intubation

- Select the proper size tube based on gestational age and weight.
- Insertion depth is weight in kilograms + 6 cm.
- Very premature neonate insertion depth is the naso-tragus distance + 1 cm.
- Provide adequate ventilation prior to attempting tube placement.
- Monitor vital signs throughout the procedure.
- Facilitate a slight neck extension prior to laryngoscope insertion while the provider is intubating the neonate.
- Tube placement is checked by auscultation and assessing for bilateral inflation and observing the tube steaming up.

- Tape the tube in place against the mouth/nose.
- Obtain an X-ray to confirm proper placement.

Lumbar Puncture

- Set up a sterile field with appropriate-sized sterile gloves for a neonatal practitioner.
- Clean the back area with an antiseptic solution.
- Obtain a lateral decubitus position by firmly rounding the shoulders and buttocks in a motion toward each other to facilitate curvature of the spine.
- The puncture is with a 22 G or 24 G needle with a stylet.
- The CSF is obtained and sent to the lab with proper labeling of the tubes.

Chest Tube Placement

- Ensure proper size of chest tube (10 Fr or 12 Fr; 10 Fr for smaller infants) and gather all equipment.
- Assist in preparing the chest area with an antiseptic solution.
- Assist as the provider makes an incision and inserts the tube, listening for a rush of air indicating that pleural penetration has occurred.
- Attach the tube to a Heimlich valve or an underwater drainage system applying negative pressure (10 to 20 cm H_2O) to the underwater drainage system.
- Once the chest tube is sutured into place, cover the incision with petroleum ointment and gauze and a clear plastic adhesive dressing.
- Obtain a chest X-ray to confirm placement.

Vascular Catheterization

Types of Catheters

- Umbilical artery catheters (UAVs)
- Peripheral artery catheters (PACs)
- Umbilical vein catheters (UVCs)
- Central venous catheters

Procedure

- Assemble the catheter tray with correct size catheter.
- Assist in obtaining measurements prior to cleansing the area with an antiseptic solution.
- The practitioner will place twill tape around the cord stump.

- The cord is stabilized with hemostats while the tip of the forceps is inserted into the vessel so dilatation can be performed.
- Once the vessel is dilated, the umbilical vessel catheter is inserted and threaded into the vessel.
- Observe for cyanosis or blanching of the leg, poor distal extremity perfusion, and hematuria.
- Measure the appropriate distance and placement by X-ray.
- Tie catheter in place using a purse-string suture with silk thread and a tape bridge to provide stability.

Abdominal Paracentesis

- Assemble equipment on a sterile field.
- Clean the lower abdomen with an antiseptic solution.
- Prepare a syringe with 1% lidocaine solution.
- Upon catheter placement, 5 to 20 cc of fluid is aspirated and the catheter is removed.
- Bandage insertion site.

Pericardiocentesis

- Prepare proper equipment tray.
- Clean the area with an antiseptic solution, including the subxiphoid area and left anterior chest.
- Obtain an ultrasound machine for sonography guidance.
- Monitor for arrhythmias throughout the procedure.
- Aspiration is continued until no additional fluid is present.
- Observe for cardiac and respiratory complications.

NEONATAL ANESTHESIA AND SURGERY

Surgery in the neonatal period is only performed when absolutely necessary. Anesthesia use carries some risks and requires careful monitoring by an experienced clinician. Commonly used anesthetic agents include inhaled anesthesia and regional anesthesia. The conditions that most commonly require surgical procedures during the neonatal period include:

- Tracheoesophageal fistula
- Gastroschisis
- Omphalocele
- Encephalocele
- Pyloric stenosis
- Congenital diaphragmatic hernia

- Imperforate anus
- Ventriculoperitoneal shunt
- Cardiac cauterization
- Posterior urethral valve excision

Consideration for Neonates Receiving Anesthesia and Undergoing Surgery

- Intraoperative fluid management
- Management of apnea
- Transitional circulation can reoccur
- Adequate ventilation during surgery
- Management of blood loss
- Maintaining glucose levels
- Temperature maintenance
- Existence of coagulopathies
- Risk of infection
- Pain management in the postoperative period
- Risk for anesthesia toxicity

References

Eichenwald, E. C., Hanen, A. R., Martin, C. R., & Stark, A. R. (2017). *Cloherty and Stark's manual of neonatal care* (8th ed.). Philadelphia, PA: Wolters Kluwer.

Ramazani, T., Shirazi, Z. H., Sarvestani, R. S., & Moiattani, M. (2014). Family-centered care in neonatal intensive care unit: A concept analysis. *International Journal of Community Based Nurse Midwifery, 2*(4), 268–278.

Westrup, B. (2015). Family-centered developmentally supportive care: The Swedish example [Soins de développement centrés sur la famille en néonatologie: Un exemple suédois]. *Archives de Pédiatrie, 22*(10), 1086–1091. doi:10.1016/j.arcped.2015.07.005

23

Management of Common NICU Complications

Respiratory, cardiovascular, and hematological issues represent the most serious and commonly occurring complications in the NICU. The nurse plays a vital role in the identification, monitoring, and management of these complications. Expertise in monitoring and ongoing assessment enables the nurse to identify changes in the newborn's condition that may warrant more intensive management strategies.

During this part of the orientation, the nurse will be able to:

1. Discuss common strategies for monitoring respiratory effort and status in the high-risk newborn.
2. Compare and contrast the different types of mechanical ventilation.
3. Delineate when to use certain types of blood products for various conditions encountered in the NICU.
4. Outline the treatment for the infant experiencing shock.

MANAGEMENT OF RESPIRATORY COMPLICATIONS

Pulmonary Function Monitoring

- Arterial blood gas monitoring

  - Collect in dried heparinized collection tubes.

- 0.2 mL sample size required
- Put collected samples on ice.

- Pulse oximetry

  - Ensure transmitter device is secured in place.

- Transcutaneous CO_2 monitoring

  - Observe probe site to assess for tissue injury.

Mechanical Ventilation

- Mechanical ventilation is complex. Different types of ventilation are selected based on the facility's available equipment, the infant's gestational age and weight, and the presence of select respiratory factors or risk factors. Adjunctive therapies may include sedation, muscle relaxation, and blood gas monitoring (Eichenwald, Hansen, Martin, & Stark, 2017).

- Continuous positive pressure (CPAP)

  - Heated humidified gas at a pressure of 3 to 8 cm H_2O with spontaneous breathing
  - Delivery via nasal mask, nasopharyngeal tube, or nasal cannula
  - Reduces need for mechanical ventilation, prevents lung injury, decreases need for surfactant, and reduces apnea
  - Not effective when frequent apnea or inadequate respiratory drive is present
  - Nasogastric tube may be necessary due to distention from swallowed air.

- High flow nasal cannula

  - Uses blended heated oxygen at >1 L/minute via nasal canula
  - Lower incidence of nasal breakdown
  - May require longer duration of assistance than CPAP
  - May be less effective than CPAP in preterm infants younger than 26 gestational weeks

- Patient-triggered, volume targeted ventilators

  - Continuous flow of heated humidified gas maintained at specified O_2 saturation level by selecting specified peak inspiratory pressure, positive end-expiratory pressure, and expiration
  - Spontaneous respiratory efforts can be made
  - Does not respond to changes in respiratory system compliance
  - If spontaneous breathing is irregular with too many breaths, infants fighting ventilation are at risk for air leak.

- Synchronized and patient-triggered ventilators

  - Often preferred ventilator for infants with some spontaneous breathing efforts
  - Measures inspiratory movement to deliver intermittent positive-pressure breaths at a fixed rate mirroring neonate's inspiratory effort and delivers a controlled rate to cover apnea episodes
  - Settings for assist-control ventilation or pressure support ventilation can be selected to reduce air leaks, reduce sedation needs, facilitate ventilator weaning, and reduce intracranial hemorrhage.
  - Observe for abnormal breath triggering due to sensor issues and artifact signaling.

- Volume-targeted ventilators

  - Patient-triggered ventilation used in infants with respiratory failure, changing lung compliance, RDS, and those receiving surfactant therapy
  - Inspiratory pressure adjusts with a specified inspiratory volume with lowest possible pressure and wide variation in V_T
  - Careful monitoring is required to detect air leaks around endotracheal tube, which can result in sensing expired rather than inspired V_Ts.

- High-frequency ventilators

  - Used an adjunctive therapy for infants on conventional ventilation
  - Ventilation achieved without large variations in lung volume
  - Improved outcomes for infants with pulmonary leak syndromes, pneumothorax, severe respiratory failure, and failure to maintain adequate ventilation on traditional ventilator
  - Different types include high-frequency oscillator (HFO), high-frequency flow interpreter (HFFI), and high-frequency jet (HFJ).
  - Provides rapid rates with V_Ts equal to dead space
  - Continuous pressure maintains elevated lung volumes
  - HFJs can deliver sigh breaths to prevent atelectasis.
  - HFFI and HFJ provides passive expiration; with HFO, expiration is controlled

- Noninvasive mechanical ventilation

  - Provides neonatal nasal intermittent positive pressure ventilation (NIPPV) that supplements CPAP

- Provides PPV without intubation and is delivered through nasal cannula
- Used in infants with apnea of prematurity, premature infants with RDS, and following extubation
- Provides inhalations to a specified peak pressure

EXTRACORPOREAL MEMBRANE OXYGENATION (ECMO)

- Modified cardiopulmonary bypass for respiratory or cardiac failure or those who failed ventilation and traditional treatment modalities.
- Provides oxygen delivery, removal of carbon dioxide, cerebral perfusion, and renal perfusion
- ECMO requires blood gas monitoring, heparin administration, administration of blood products, conditions, antibiotic therapy, administration of Amicar, sedation, pain control, intravenous fluids, lipid administration, and ultrafilter placement.
- Obtain head ultrasound prior and during ECMO.
- Obtain serial EEGs if seizures are detected.
- Assess for mechanical problems including clots in the circuit, cannula issues, oxygenator failure, tubing issues, poor catheter position, excessive catheter length, and improper pump position.
- Assess for signs and symptoms of hypovolemia, pneumothorax, tamponade, vasodilatation, arrhythmia, intracranial hemorrhage, renal failure, and pulmonary embolism.
- Ensure pump is placed at level of head and not above the head.
- Ventilator settings allow lungs to rest yet remain slightly inflated to prevent collapse.
- Conditioning cycles challenge the patient by allowing reduced settings while monitoring gas exchange.
- Decannulation is considered when the infant can be supported on a ventilator device.

MANAGEMENT OF CARDIOVASCULAR AND HEMATOLOGICAL CONDITIONS

Administration of Blood Products

- Blood products are administered for poor oxygenation or coagulation defects. Blood products undergo irradiation and leukoreduction as a means of combatting transmission of infectious agents. Many families request directed donor blood transfusion. Direct donor blood is associated with higher infection rates, maternal antibody exposure, and risk of an immune response to human leukocyte antigen.

Types of Blood Products

- Packed red blood cells (PRBCs)

  - Used when signs and symptoms of hypoxia are present or exchange transfusions are warranted
  - Side effects may include
    - Acute hemolytic reactions
    - Allergic reactions
    - Volume overload
    - Hypocalcemia
    - Hypothermia
    - Transfusion-associated acute lung injury
    - Hyperkalemia
    - Febrile nonhemolytic reactions
    - Bacterial contamination
    - Transfusion-associated-graft-versus-host disease (TA-GvHD)

- Fresh frozen and thawed plasma

  - Used to treat coagulopathies
  - Acute hemolytic reactions rarely occur.
  - Ensure products are compatible with patient's blood group to prevent antibody incompatibilities.
  - Infuse transfusions slowly to prevent citrate-induced hypocalcemia.

- Platelets

  - Use in preterm infants shown to rescue intracranial hemorrhage
  - Increased risk of bacterial contamination
  - Removal of plasma reduces ABO incompatibility issues

- Granulocytes

  - May be used with severe neutropenia, abnormal neutrophil production, or infection not responding to antibiotic therapy
  - Must be transfused within 24 hours of collection
  - Observe for pulmonary signs and symptoms.

- Whole blood

  - Used in exchange transfusions and ECMO in some situations
  - Maximum shelf life is 7 days

- Intravenous immunoglobin

  - Primary component is immunoglobin G
  - Administered for alloimmune disorders or immunoglobin deficiency syndromes
  - May use hyperimmune immunoglobulins for varicella zoster or RSV
  - Observe for tachycardia and hypertension during and immediately following administration.

- Umbilical cord blood

  - Collected from cord blood at the time of birth; tested, and frozen for later use
  - Used as autologous transplants
  - Febrile reactions more common
  - Irradiation cannot be performed.

NEONATAL SHOCK

Infant Risk Factors

- Very-low-birth-weight infants
- Perinatal depression
- Septic shock
- Preterm infants with PDAS
- Preterm infants with pressor-resistant hypotension

Common Causes

- Low vascular tone
- Hypovolemic shock
- Decreased cardiac functioning
- Restricted blood flow
- Inadequate oxygenation

Symptoms of Shock

- Pallor and cold skin
- Delayed capillary refill time
- Tachycardia and narrow pulse pressure, weak peripheral pulses
- Ileus
- Oliguria
- Lethargy
- Change in consciousness
- Hypotension
- Preterm infants are at a greater risk for intracranial hemorrhage and PVL and neurological injury.

Treatment

- Intravenous fluids
- Corrections of etiological factors
- Calcium administration
- CVP monitoring

Medications

- Inotropes (dopamine, dobutamine, epinephrine, and milrinone)
- Vasopressors (dopamine, vasopressin, and hydrocortisone replacement)

Reference

Eichenwald, E. C., Hanen, A. R., Martin, C. R., & Stark, A. R. (2017). *Cloherty and Stark's manual of neonatal care* (8th ed.). Philadelphia, PA: Wolters Kluwer.

24

Neonatal Ethical Conflicts and Considerations

In the United States, there are almost 4 million births each year. Of these, 2.7% (15,000/year) will have birth defects incompatible with life. Critically fragile newborns are at a lifetime risk for adverse outcomes and disabilities. Parents may be faced with the option of making complicated decisions regarding the continuation of pregnancy in these circumstances. The nurse provides support and education when a family is facing the death of an infant. Perinatal hospice can provide support, neonatal care, and comfort measures for dying newborns.

During this part of the orientation, the nurse will be able to:

1. Delineate the factors that need to be considered when making decisions on the care of neonates born on the threshold of viability.
2. Delineate the adverse outcomes associated with critically fragile neonates.
3. Analyze the needs of families following a neonatal death.
4. Describe the purpose of perinatal hospice care.
5. List ethical resources that are available for care providers involved in ethical decision-making.

INFANTS BORN ON THE THRESHOLD OF VIABILITY

The threshold of viability takes into account gestational age at the time of birth and birth weight. The combination of these factors can drastically affect morbidity and mortality (Tables 24.1 and 24.2). Infants on the threshold of viability make up less than 1% of all births in the United States, but account for 47% of neonatal deaths (Haug et al., 2018). Although these infants may survive, they are at risk for long-term disabilities, including:

- Psychomotor disabilities
- Neuromuscular disabilities
- Mental disabilities
- Sensory disabilities
- Communication-related disabilities
- Cerebral palsy

Table 24.1

Survival Rates Associated With Completed Gestational Weeks	
Completed Gestational Weeks	Survival Rate (%)
21	0
22	21
23	30
24	50
25	75
26	80
27	90
>28	>90

Source: Data from Lemons, J. A., Bauer, C. R., Oh, W., Korones, S. B., Papile, L. A., Stoll, B. J., . . . Stevenson, D. K. (2001). Very low birth weight outcomes of the National Institute of Child health and human development neonatal research network, January 1995 through December 1996. NICHD Neonatal Research Network. *Pediatrics, 107*(1), E1. doi:10.1542/peds.107.1.e1

Table 24.2

Infant Survival by Birth Weight	
Birth Weight (g)	Survival Rate (%)
400–500	11
501–600	31

(continued)

Table 24.2

Infant Survival by Birth Weight (*continued*)	
Birth Weight (g)	**Survival Rate (%)**
601–700	62
701–800	75
801–900	88
901–1,000	90
>1,000	>92

Source: Data from Lemons, J. A., Bauer, C. R., Oh, W., Korones, S. B., Papile, L. A., Stoll, B. J., . . . Stevenson, D. K. (2001). Very low birth weight outcomes of the National Institute of Child health and human development neonatal research network, January 1995 through December 1996. NICHD Neonatal Research Network. *Pediatrics, 107*(1), E1. doi:10.1542/peds.107.1.e1

Outcomes Associated With Critically Fragile Neonates

Newborns weighing between 500 and 750 g are at risk for the following adverse outcomes:

- Growth failure
- Intraventricular hemorrhage
- Respiratory distress syndrome
- Chronic lung disease
- Severe brain injury (intraventricular hemorrhage and periventricular leukomalacia)
- Necrotizing enterocolitis
- Nosocomial infections
- Retinopathy of prematurity
- Cerebral palsy
- Vision impairment
- Hearing loss

Evaluating Infant Status at Birth

Newborns born on the threshold of viability should be assessed and care decisions should be made based on the following:

- Gestational age
- Birth weight
- Condition at time of birth
- Morbidity and mortality data and statistics
- Newborn's response to resuscitative and stabilizing measures
- Parental preferences

- Knowledge that care plan may change based on newborn's condition
- Withdrawal of life support may be warranted if deterioration of condition occurs

DECISION TO TRANSITION TO COMFORT CARE MEASURES

The decision not to pursue aggressive life-saving measures is difficult to determine. In some cases, clear guidelines inform care and decision-making. In other circumstances, there is more of a gray area. Many facilities lack clear policies and procedures to aid in the provision of comfort measures. In these circumstances, standardized orders, physician and staff education to support the grieving family, and use of an interdisciplinary team to provide support and services should be a standard of care. Transition to comfort measures is appropriate when any of the following circumstances are present:

- Irreversibly comatose
- Treatment is only prolonging death
- Treatment is futile for survival

Fast Facts

In 1995, neonatal care guidelines became law under the Federal Child Abuse Law.

NEWBORNS WITH LETHAL ANOMALIES

Anomalies not compatible with life will result in newborn death. Of infants born with lethal anomalies, 75% will die within 10 days of life, with 90% dying within 4 months of birth. Diagnosis of lethal anomalies typically occurs during the prenatal period, although the possibility of a missed diagnosis or lack of prenatal care may lead to undetected anomalies not identified until birth. Routine prenatal tools that typically identify these anomalies include:

- First-trimester screening (ultrasound examination for nuchal translucency testing with maternal blood screening)
- Ultrasound
- Chronic villus sampling
- Amniocentesis
- Fetal echocardiography
- Quadruple screen

Types of Birth Defects Considered Lethal Anomalies

Lethal anomalies are those that are considered incompatible with life. The most common defects include:

- Anencephaly
- Trisomy 13
- Trisomy 18
- Renal agenesis
- Thanatophoric dysplasia
- Alobar holoprosencephaly
- Certain types of hydrocephalic cases
- Certain hypoplastic cardiac conditions (when heart transplant is not a treatment option)

Pregnancy Options for Birth Defects Incompatible With Life

When a lethal birth defect is identified, extensive counseling is warranted. Families are generally given the following pregnancy options:

- Continuation of pregnancy in a supportive manner with no planned life-saving interventions at birth
- Continuation of pregnancy with life-saving measures provided at birth
- Elective termination of pregnancy

The following care measures are imperative:

- Complete explanation of diagnosis, prognosis, and anticipated outcomes
- Referral to genetic specialist/perinatologist
- Discussion of each pregnancy option
- Information that infants with the identified diagnosis have rarely survived
- Communication of life expectancy averages
- Honest prognosis of surviving infants with vast medical complications
- Assistance with second opinion per parent request
- Risk of reoccurrence with future pregnancies
- Referral to child life specialist to help with sibling preparation
- Bereavement support and planning (should begin at time of diagnosis)

Fast Facts

Although online resources can provide support and valuable information, "miracles" posted on blogs and other sites can lead to unreasonable expectations and further pain.

Nursing Care to Families Facing a Birth Defect Incompatible With Life

Care measures include holistic care based on the selected pregnancy option. Each family needs specific, individualized, holistic nursing care regardless of the pregnancy option they choose.

Continuation of Pregnancy

Continuation of a pregnancy following prenatal diagnosis of a lethal anomaly occurs in 18% of women (Haug et al., 2018). Appropriate care measures are needed to ensure supportive, family-centered care, including:

- Ongoing prenatal care with a perinatologist
- Frequent ultrasound monitoring
- Monitoring for maternal complications
- Referral for counseling and psychological support
- Family support, including support groups and peer support
- Preparation on expectations of infant appearance, birth process, and anticipated outcomes at the time of birth
- Assistance with sibling education and support
- Assistance with a detailed birth plan based on the family's preferences

  - Desired interventions/lack of interventions at the time of birth
  - Identification of support persons to be present during labor and birth
  - Postbirth family/sibling visitation
  - Planned newborn interactions following live birth

    - Holding infant
    - Breastfeeding infant
    - Dressing newborn
    - Sibling/extended family member visit
    - Spending time with the infant alone
    - Pain control for newborn

  - Desired interaction with newborn following death

    - Holding infant
    - Keeping infant at the bedside for a certain period of time
    - Visit from extended family/siblings
    - Religious ceremonies

  - Predetermined plan on notifying friends/family of birth outcomes after delivery
  - Postdelivery support plan

- Clergy
- Support groups
- Funeral home arrangements

- Memory box
- Consultation with a grief counselor
- Contingency plan of care for newborns who exceed the expected life expectancy period
- Plan of care with life expectancies more than several days

  - Discharge home
  - Palliative care
  - Perinatal hospice referral

- Autopsy
- Assist with identifying resources for final arrangements

Fast Facts

Families that make comprehensive plans for the newborn's birth and death feel a sense of control during the labor, birth, and post-partum periods. Creating a detailed birth, life, and death plan can empower parents during this time of intense grief.

Termination of Pregnancy

- Method of termination is dependent on gestational age at time of termination
- Education on procedure, expectations, and appearance of infant following delivery
- Psychological support
- Birth plan

  - Presence of support persons
  - Postbirth interaction with infant

    - Holding infant
    - Dressing infant
    - Photos
    - Visitation of extended family members
    - Support persons, including clergy, grief counselor

  - Autopsy and final arrangements

- Assist with identifying resources for final arrangements

Parents should be counseled to use caution with how much information is shared with others and limit specific information sharing to friends and family who will offer support and acceptance. Discordant opinions can cause pain, guilt, and additional stress.

NEWBORN DEATH AND DYING

Each year, 19,000 newborns die in the neonatal period. The leading causes of neonatal death include:

- Premature birth
- Congenital heart defects
- Lung defects
- Chromosomal/genetic defects
- Brain and central nervous system defects

Perinatal Hospice (HRC)

"Perinatal hospice is a philosophy of family-centered care that addresses the expectations and intentions of families who choose to continue a pregnancy after their baby is diagnosed with a life-limiting condition. It includes the broad goals of palliative care: to anticipate, prevent, and relieve suffering (physical, psychological, and spiritual), to preserve dignity, and to promote quality of life for baby and family, while honoring parental preferences and wishes for their baby's care regardless of length of life" (Limbo, Toce, & Peck, 2016, p. 1). Palliative perinatal care services involve an intradisciplinary team that provides seamless care throughout the pregnancy, termination (if this is chosen), intrapartum, and postpartum period. The following should be provided:

- Seamless communication among care team members is essential.
- Bereavement services should be threaded throughout each stage of the pregnancy through the postpartum period.
- Parental, cultural, religious, family, and personal beliefs should provide a foundation for care planning and developing a birth plan.

- Palliative care services should be coordinated among interdisciplinary team members and sites of care (outpatient prenatal service site, hospital facility, outpatient services, home care services).
- Components of care should include a formal prenatal consultation; creation of a detailed birth plan; and access and consultation to neonatal and pediatric specialists.
- A case manager should be appointed to guide care and advise the family that differences of opinion may occur, especially if the prenatal diagnosis and postbirth expectations vary greatly.

ETHICAL RESOURCES FOR HEALTH PROFESSIONALS

In some cases, there may be more of a gray area or circumstances where physicians/care providers and parents are in disagreement about whether to pursue aggressive therapies or to transition to comfort measures. In these cases, utilize the following resources:

- Identify an independent advocate for the newborn.
- Consult the state's child protection agency to provide jurisdiction for decision-making.
- Consult the Infant Care Review Committees (Infant Bioethics Committees) to assist in and guiding complex decisions.
- Obtain expert consultation from an ethicist with expertise in neonatology.

References

Haug, S., Farooqi, S., Wilson, C. G., Hopper, A., Oei, G., & Carter, B. (2018). Survey on neonatal end-of-life comfort care guidelines across America. *Journal of Pain and Symptom Management, 55*(3), 979–984.

Lemons, J. A., Bauer, C. R., Oh, W., Korones, S. B., Papile, L. A., Stoll, B. J., . . . Stevenson, D. K. (2001). Very low birth weight outcomes of the National Institute of Child health and human development neonatal research network, January 1995 through December 1996. NICHD Neonatal Research Network. *Pediatrics, 107*(1), E1. doi:10.1542/peds.107.1.e1

Limbo, R., Toce, S., & Peck, T. (2016). *Resolve through sharing (RTS) position paper on perinatal palliative care* (Rev. Ed.). La Crosse, WI: Gundersen Lutheran Medical Foundation, Inc.

VIII

Discharge and Parent Teaching

25

Discharge Teaching for Parents

For new parents, leaving the healthcare setting can create mixed feelings. Parents need extensive teaching prior to discharge in order to learn how to adequately and safely provide for their newborn. Ongoing well-baby visits and immunizations are imperative for the newborn to ensure proper growth, development, and optimal health.

During this part of the orientation, the nurse will be able to:

1. Identify appropriate components of discharge from the neonatal intensive care unit (NICU) setting.
2. List the appropriate intervals for routine well-baby visits during the first month of life.
3. Discuss strategies to reduce parental refusal of immunizations.

DISCHARGE FROM THE NICU SETTING

Discharge from the NICU setting can bring a variety of emotions for new parents who may be both anxious and excited at the prospect of caring for their baby at home. Components of discharge planning should include:

■ Encourage rooming-in prior to discharge so parents know the infant's schedule and needs.

- Ensure that a follow-up appointment with an outpatient provider has been scheduled.
- Affirm that a car seat safety test was performed for infants born prior to 35 gestational weeks.
- Confirm completion of CPR class by parents or caregivers.
- Provide appropriate education on:
  - Feeding
  - Monitoring weight gain
  - Proper sleep positioning
  - Vaccination schedules
  - Proper medication administration
  - Other pertinent medical or infant care information

- If being discharged on medications:
  - Review medication.
  - Discuss the purpose, dosage, frequency, duration of use, and route of medication.
  - Cover what to do if infant vomits medication, and other components of medication administration.
  - Discharge with prescriptions and ensure medications are available at designated pharmacies prior to discharge.

- Ensure the household can adequately handle the electrical needs of any monitoring or medical equipment.
  - Teach proper use of medical or monitoring equipment prior to discharge.

- Discuss with parents who they would like present at home after discharge (if they would like to avoid visitors, discuss notification strategies prior to discharge).
- Review needed supplies and equipment with parents prior to discharge.
- Obtain Hepatitis B consent and vaccination prior to discharge.
- Obtain the RSV consent and vaccination prior to discharge between October and April.
- Complete the newborn hearing screening.
- Ensure that a car seat was installed prior to arrival at hospital.
- Ensure that an outfit and blanket was brought for the ride home.
- Take the discharge summary sheet home to take to the pediatrician appointment.
- Provide access to videos, written resources, brochures, pamphlets, apps, and discharge information.

INITIAL PEDIATRIC FOLLOW-UP VISIT FOLLOWING NICU DISCHARGE

The initial follow-up visit following a NICU stay has many of the components of a well-baby visit.

- NICU babies to be seen within 24 to 48 hours of discharge to establish care with an outpatient provider.
- Some facilities offer specialized clinics for infants who were previously admitted to the NICU.
- Depending on the current health status, the infant may see a nurse practitioner, physician's assistant, pediatrician, or developmental pediatrician.
- Infants with specific health needs may warrant follow-up with medical specialists related to specific medical issues or complications.
- Infants with suspected or known developmental delays should receive an early intervention consult.
- Collaborate with a case manager for home health, early intervention services, and medical equipment needs.
- Assess to determine the need for physical therapy, occupational therapy, speech therapy (swallowing and feeding specialists).
- Refer to specialized NICU parent support groups.
- Assess mother for postpartum mood and anxiety disorders (PMADs), which are more common in women with children with NICU stays and adverse health conditions.
- Administer vaccinations (or develop a schedule for vaccinations).

WELL-BABY VISITS

Components of well-baby visits include examination and evaluation of the following:

- Weight
- Length
- Abdominal circumference
- Head circumference
- Evaluation of appropriate growth and development
- Physical examination
- Parental education

  - Safety
  - Ongoing identification of risk factors
  - Risk-reduction strategies
  - Health-promotion strategies

Although the outpatient newborn exam typically occurs within 2 to 5 days after birth, parents should be taught to seek medical attention earlier if a complication or unexpected event occurs.

Newborn Examinations

The newborn should be seen within 2 to 5 days of birth (Table 25.1) and again between 1 and 4 weeks. Essential components of those visits should include evaluation of the following:

Table 25.1

Assessment Data and Parent Teaching for Newborn Well Visits		
Age	Age-Specific Assessment Data	Parent Teaching
2–5 days	■ Weight loss/gain/presence of abnormal vomiting or other gastrointestinal issues ■ Infant feeding method ■ Frequency of voiding and stooling ■ Safety measures being used (not leaving infant unattended where falls could occur, leaving infant with appropriate caretakers, providing infant with appropriate nutrition, ensuring safe environment free from environmental hazards) ■ Volume of milk consumption to determine whether vitamin D supplementation is needed ■ Use of infant care seat and current position ■ Sleep positions ■ Smoke/carbon monoxide detectors in home ■ Hepatitis B vaccination status	■ Normal newborn growth and development ■ Breastfeeding frequency/duration ■ Problems/concerns related to breastfeeding ■ Pumping and breast milk storage ■ Safety issues related to formula preparation ■ Safe sleeping positions ("Back to Sleep" positioning) ■ Normal infant sleep patterns ■ Crying patterns ■ Safety issues (fall prevention, possible choking risks, suffocation hazards, car seat use, safe water temperature) ■ Participation in an infant cardiopulmonary resuscitation course ■ Assess for maternal postpartum depression and mood disorders ■ Abusive head trauma (AHT) ■ Illness prevention/handwashing ■ Prevention of AHT ■ Importance of immunizations ■ Sunburn prevention

(continued)

Table 25.1

Assessment Data and Parent Teaching for Newborn Well Visits (*continued*)		
Age	**Age-Specific Assessment Data**	**Parent Teaching**
1–4 weeks	■ Feeding difficulties ■ Inadequate weight gain ■ Cord condition/cord site	■ Crying/colic ■ Bathing ■ Illness prevention/handwashing ■ Car safety ■ Ways to soothe baby ■ Prevention of AHT ■ Future immunizations ■ Sunburn prevention

- Evaluation of feeding
- Weight gain/loss
- Adjustment to parenthood
- Identification of specific parental concerns
- Safety

The hepatitis B immunization is generally given prior to discharge from the medical facility. Infant immunizations typically begin at 2 months; however, education on the importance of immunizations should begin at the initial newborn visits. For families traveling out of the country, the Centers for Disease Control and Prevention (CDC) recommends certain immunizations.

Family and Environmental Risk Factors

Assess certain risk factors that can put the infant at risk for adverse health outcomes:

- Family risk factors

  - History of intimate partner violence or domestic violence
  - History of past child abuse or child neglect
  - Low level of parental education achievement
  - Low socioeconomic status/poverty
  - Adolescent parents
  - Severe parental mental illness
  - Parental substance abuse
  - Parents who oppose/decline immunizations
  - Presence of stressful life events within the family
  - Low parental IQ
  - Lack of maternal–infant attachment

- Environmental risk factors
  - Lack of family/community support
  - Lack of access to health care
  - Rural geographic location
  - Crowded living conditions
  - Exposure to secondhand smoke
  - Enrollment in low-quality child care

Fast Facts

Infants exposed to secondhand smoke are more likely to experience allergies, asthma, and hospitalizations during the first year of life.

Well visits should be scheduled at regular intervals:

- 2 to 5 days after birth
- 1 to 4 weeks
- 2 months
- 4 months
- 6 months
- 9 months
- 12 months

Immunizations

Immunizations can dramatically reduce childhood and community illness. Immunizations begin at birth (hepatitis B) and continue throughout childhood. Appendix A includes the CDC vaccination guidelines.

Recommended Immunizations for Overseas Travel

Infants traveling outside of the United States are particularly vulnerable to infectious diseases because of their immature immune systems and lack of adequate vaccinations due to their young age. Overseas travel requires preplanning and specific interventions to ensure infant safety. Parents should be advised to:

- Consult a travel immunization specialist to determine which specific vaccines are needed for the country of travel.

- Consult the pediatrician 3 to 4 months ahead of travel to initiate an accelerated vaccine schedule.
- If possible, travel should be delayed until the infant is 9 months of age, when a yellow fever vaccine can be given.
- All infants should receive a meningococcal meningitis vaccine prior to any overseas travel.
- Counsel parents that some vaccines cannot be given early.
- Breastfeeding is the safest feeding choice.
- If formula is used, parents should bring formula with them and only use purified water to mix the formula.

Parental Refusal of Immunizations

Approximately 6% of parents refuse vaccinations, whereas another 13% delay vaccinations (Davidson, Ladewig, & London, 2020). Parents refuse or delay immunizations for a number of reasons (Figure 25.1):

- Belief that diseases vaccines guard against have been eradicated
- Concerns over vaccine safety
- Belief that multiple vaccines overload the immune system
- Belief that vaccines are associated with autism
- Belief that ingredients found in vaccines (thimerosal and aluminum salts) are dangerous
- Belief that the medical condition their child has makes vaccinations dangerous
- Personal, philosophical, or religious beliefs

Counseling for Parents Refusing Immunizations

- Begin discussing vaccination information at the initial visit.
- Provide factual information in a respectful, nonpatronizing, and nonconfrontational manner.
- Provide vaccination information sheets at least 1 month prior to the scheduled immunization.
- Discuss the need to prevent community outbreaks.
- Direct parents to credible websites.
- Be respectful of parents' authority. (Davidson et al., 2020)

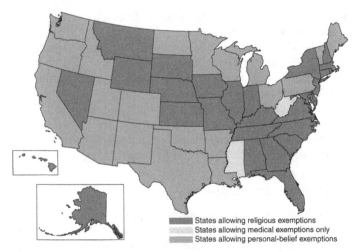

Figure 25.1 State exemption status for immunizations.

Source: Centers for Disease Control and Prevention. (2013). *State vaccination requirements*. Retrieved from http://www.cdc.gov/vaccines/imz-managers/laws/index.html

- Provide sucrose administration and swaddling as pain reduction mechanisms during injections.
- Ongoing refusal warrants appropriate interactions.
  - Complete of the American Academy of Pediatrics Refusal-to-Vaccinate form.
  - Notify the parents of office/clinic policies if refusal warrants patient dismissal from practice.

References

Davidson, M. R., Ladewig, P. L., & London, M. L. (2020). *Old's maternal newborn nursing and women's health across the lifespan*. Boston, MA: Pearson Education.

26

Newborn Care

Newborn care is a major concern for new parents. The nurse plays a critical role in providing education and demonstrating newborn care practices to new parents. New parents may be unfamiliar with normal care practices, when to seek medical care, normal newborn sleeping, and crying behaviors. The nurse provides education so parents can know what to expect and when to call a healthcare provider if medical issues arise after discharge.

During this part of the orientation, the nurse will be able to:

1. Provide a demonstration of a newborn bath.
2. Review signs and symptoms of infection with the umbilical cord that warrant medical intervention.
3. Discuss newborn urinary and stooling patterns.
4. Differentiate between newborn sleep and wake cycles.
5. Outline reasons for crying in the newborn period.

BATHING

Bathing in the newborn period should begin with sponge bathing until the umbilical cord falls off completely. Sponge bathing can be performed every 2 to 3 days, or more frequently in summer months as needed. Parents should be taught the following for sponge bathing:

- Obtain all supplies prior to starting the bath (washcloth, towels, soap).
- Place the infant on a surface that can support the infant and hold supplies.
- Never leave the infant unattended during bath.
- Obtain a bowl of water.
- Undress the infant and keep him or her covered with a towel to prevent heat loss.
- Use a small amount of mild cleanser that is free of fragrance and dye, tearless, and pH neutral.
- Dry each body area to prevent heat loss.
- Never hold an infant under running water, as temperature changes can occur.
- Review a systematic method for bathing, starting with the eyes, face, and progressing downward.
- The genitals should be cleaned last, prior to washing the hair.
- Once the body has been bathed, infants can be swaddled so hair can be washed.

TUB BATHS AND SHOWERING

- Tub baths should not be started until the umbilical cord has completely fallen off.
- Obtain all needed equipment.
- Test water to ensure proper temperature prior to placing the infant in the tub.
- Support of the head and body is needed.
- Never leave a child unattended to answer the phone, door, check on other children, etc.
- Parents wishing to shower infants during their own shower should be counseled on safety issues.
- Newborns should never be taken into hot tubs or saunas due to extreme temperatures.

Fast Facts

Many new parents are anxious about giving their newborn a bath. Providing a demonstration allows the parents to engage in the process and ask questions. Alternatively, some facilities offer newborn bathing classes on the unit in a group setting where teaching is targeted for groups of new parents.

SKIN AND NAIL CARE

- Never cut nails in the hospital setting prior to discharge due to the risk of nosocomial infection.
- Parents may file or cut nails with infant-sized nail clippers.
- Cutting nails after a bath can soften nails.
- If the skin is nicked or cut during trimming, keep the area clean and watch for signs of infection (uncommon).
- Baby powder should never be used because the particles can cause respiratory issues.
- Lotion and creams are generally not needed; if used, one designed for infants should be used sparingly.
- Avoid direct sunlight and damaging rays; keep baby in a shaded area or in a stroller.
- If absolutely necessary, apply a small amount of SPF 30 sunscreen after testing on the wrist prior to application.

CORD CARE AND ASSESSMENT

- Cords typically continue to dry for 7 to 21 days before falling off.
- A small wound may be present at the site and will heal within a few days.
- The cord should be kept clean and dry.
- Diapers should be folded underneath the cord.
- One-piece outfits should be avoided until the cord falls off.
- Signs of infection warrant immediate evaluation

  - Fever
  - The cord or surrounding area becomes red, warm, or edematous
  - Foul-smelling odor from cord
  - Pus
  - Active bleeding

- Umbilical granulomas (areas that do not heal) should be reported to the pediatrician.

MAINTAINING AN APPROPRIATE THERMAL ENVIRONMENT AT HOME

- The temperature setting should be between 68°F to 72°F in the winter and 75°F to 78°F in the summer.
- Avoid fans, drafty areas, open windows, and direct access to heat/air conditioning sources.

- Do not overbundle/overdress the newborn, as this increases the risk of sudden infant death syndrome.
- Sleep in a light-weight, single-layer item that would be comfortable for an adult in the same room
- The infant should not feel hot to touch or be perspiring profusely.
- In higher temperatures, the baby requires increased fluid consumption to prevent dehydration.
- In colder temperatures, extra layers may be needed to prevent chilling.

TEMPERATURE VARIATIONS AND SYMPTOMS RELATED TO ILLNESS

- A normal temperature is 97°F to 100.3°F (rectal).
- The presence of a fever or low temperature can indicate infection.
- Fevers in newborns and infants younger than 3 months are cause for concern.
- Lethargy is an important sign of illness.

REASONS TO SEEK MEDICAL ATTENTION

- Fever exceeds 100.4°F in newborn/infant less than 3 months
- Lethargy
- Refusal to feed
- Cough
- Signs of an earache (pulling on ear)
- Unusual fussiness or sleepiness
- Vomiting
- Diarrhea (more than 1 occurrence per hour, blood in the stool)
- Hard stools with straining and no bowel movement for 3 days
- Seizures
- Fewer than four wet diapers per day
- Dehydration (dry mouth, fewer than four wet diapers/day, sunken soft spot, lack of tears, irritability)
- More than two green watery stools in a 24-hour period

Fast Facts

Parents should be encouraged to call their healthcare provider immediately when in doubt regarding an illness in their newborn. Stress to parents that it is better to call and receive reassurance than not call and have a critical emergency occur.

NORMAL URINARY AND STOOLING PATTERNS

- Infants should void within 24 hours of birth.
- After 10 days, colorless, odorless urine is excreted up to 15 times per day.
- Initially, multiple stools are excreted each day.
- After 2 weeks of age, stooling may become less frequent.
- Breastfed infants tend to have multiple loose, mustard-colored stools with a sour-milk smell several times each day.
- Formula-fed infants tend to have brown, semi-formed stools that are firm and pasty with a foul odor, which can occur every day to every other day.
- Grunting or turning red during stooling is normal and not a sign of constipation.
- Constipation is marked by hard stools and straining.
- Diarrhea stools are frequent, loose, and watery and may result in a foul-smelling odor.

NORMAL NEWBORN SLEEP HABITS

- Newborns sleep a total of 16 to 17 hours per day.
- Newborns sleep for periods of 2 to 4 hours at a time.
- There is an increase in time spent in rapid eye movement (REM) sleep, which is lighter and more easily disturbed.
- At 2 weeks of age, begin distinguishing night and day and encouraging nighttime sleeping.

  - Keep active when awake during the day.
  - Keep rooms brightly lit.
  - Wake for all feedings.
  - Do not attempt to reduce normal household noise.
  - At night, do not wake for feedings,
  - Do not engage in play or talk excessively with newborn at night.
  - Keep lights dim and the room quiet.
  - Put back to sleep after each feeding.
  - Establish bedtime rituals (changing into night clothes, singing, kissing goodnight).

- Never administer over-the-counter or home remedies for sleeping.

INFANT SLEEP–WAKE CYCLES

The normal infant goes through a series of sleep and wake states on a regular basis. These states are marked by specific physical characteristics, physical activities, and responses. By being aware of the normal resources, caregivers can gauge the newborn's state so feeding, interactions, and care needs can be accomplished. Table 26.1 shows the various newborn sleep–wake cycles.

Table 26.1

Infant Sleep–Wake Cycles

Newborn State	Physical Characteristics	Physical Activity and Responses	Caregiver Implications
Quiet sleep (also known as deep sleep)	Anabolic, restorative sleep, increased cell mitosis and replication, lowered oxygen consumption, release of growth hormone.	Typically still but may occasionally startle or twitch. May have occasional sucking movements. Slow and regular breathing pattern. Only intense or disturbing stimuli will arouse baby. Threshold to stimuli is high.	Difficult to arouse for feedings. Teach parents to time feedings when baby is in a more responsive state. Baby may arouse slightly if an attempt is made to awaken but typically returns to the quiet sleep state.
Active sleep (also known as light sleep or rapid eye movement [REM] state)	Processing and recording information. Often linked to learning. Is the highest proportion of sleep and precedes awakening.	Some body movements occur. Rapid eye movement (REM), closed eyelids may flutter. May smile or make fussing or crying noises. Irregular breathing is common. More responsive to internal stimuli (hunger) and external stimuli (such as being picked up by caregiver). When stimulated may arouse, return to quiet sleep, or remain in active sleep.	Inexperienced care providers may attempt to feed when baby makes normal crying sounds.

(continued)

Table 26.1

Infant Sleep-Wake Cycles (*continued*)

Newborn State	Physical Characteristics	Physical Activity and Responses	Caregiver Implications
Drowsy (also known as semi-dozing)	May return to sleep or awaken further.	Smooth movements with variable activity level. May experience mild startles intermittently. Eyes may open and close. May appear heavy lidded, or eyes may appear like slits. May have no facial movements and appear still, or may have some facial movements. Irregular breathing. Slowed reactions to stimuli. May change to other states such as quiet alert, active alert, or crying.	To stimulate baby, provide verbal, sight, or oral stimulation. If left alone, baby may return to a sleep state.
Quiet alert	Attentive to environment, focus attention on stimuli.	Minimal body activity. Eyes open and bright. Attentive appearance. Regular breathing. Most attentive focus on stimuli.	In the first hours after birth, may experience intense alertness before going into a long sleeping period. This state increases in intensity as the baby becomes older. Providing stimuli will help maintain a quiet alert or active alert state. Baby provides pleasure and positive feedback to care providers. Good time to feed baby.

(*continued*)

Table 26.1

Infant Sleep-Wake Cycles (*continued*)			
Newborn State	**Physical Characteristics**	**Physical Activity and Responses**	**Caregiver Implications**
Active alert	Baby's eyes are open, not as bright as in quiet alert. More body activity than in a quiet alert state.	Smooth movements may be interspersed with mild startles from time to time. Eyes open with a gazed, dull appearance. Facial movements may be still with or without movement. Reacts to stimuli with delayed responses to stimuli, or may change to quiet alert or crying state.	Baby may be fussy and become sensitive to stimuli, and may become more and more active and start crying. If fatigue or caregiver interventions disturb this state, baby may return to a drowsy or sleep state.
Crying	Communication tool, response to unpleasant stimuli from environment or internal stimuli. Characterized by intense crying for more than 15 seconds.	Increased motor activity, skin color changes to darkened appearance, red, or ruddy. Eyes may be tightly closed or open. Facial grimaces may occur. Breathing may be more irregular than in other states. Very responsive to internal or external unpleasant stimuli.	Indicates that the baby's limits have been reached. May be able to console self and return to an alert or sleep state, or may need intervention from caregiver.

Source: Data from Davidson, M. R., Ladewig, P. L., & London, M. L. (2020). *Old's maternal newborn nursing and women's health across the lifespan.* Boston, MA: Pearson Education.

CRYING BEHAVIORS

- Vary from infant to infant, from virtually none to frequent crying episodes
- Increase at about 2 weeks after birth
- Peak at 6 weeks
- Decrease gradually until stable at 3 to 4 months of age
- One fussy period per day is common

Common Causes for Crying

- Hunger
- Gastrointestinal reflux disease
- Flatus
- Food intolerances in maternal diet associated with breastfeeding
- Colic
- Illness

Interventions for Parents of Crying Newborns

- Respond quickly to crying.
- Look for hunger cues (awake state, lip-smacking, rooting, putting hands in the mouth).
- Breastfeed baby on demand.
- Burp newborn after feeding.
- Place over your lap on abdomen and gently rub back.
- Check environmental factors to rule out whether the newborn is too hot or too cold.
- Assess for fever, lethargy, and signs of illness.
- Change diaper.
- Encourage sleep.
- Avoid letting the infant become overtired.
- Carrying and holding newborns reduces crying.

Reference

Davidson, M. R., Ladewig, P. L., & London, M. L. (2020). *Old's maternal newborn nursing and women's health across the lifespan* (11th ed.). Boston, MA: Pearson Education.

IX

Promoting Healthy Families in the Community

27

Home Environment and Infant Safety

Promotion of health and wellness for the newborn and infant begins immediately following birth and continues into the first year of life. Nurses play a crucial role in providing parental education about infant injury and illness prevention. By identifying at-risk parents, additional support and interventions can be implemented to support families with limited resources.

During this part of the orientation, the nurse will be able to:

1. Identify risk factors in the home that can result in infant injury.
2. Discuss components of home safety that can be utilized to protect the childbearing family from environmental risks.
3. Review the principles of a proper thermal environment.
4. Describe the importance of performing an environmental risk assessment.

SAFETY IN THE HOME SETTING

The importance of home safety cannot be stressed enough. A safe home environment safeguards the infant from risk and harm. There are multiple environmental factors that can predispose infants and young children to harm in the home setting. Review components of safety within the home environment with all new parents.

Smoke Alarm

- The installation of smoke alarms is recommended in each bedroom, outside each sleeping area, and on each level of the home, including the basement.
- Smoke alarms installed in kitchens should be 10 feet away from a cooking appliance to minimize false alarms. Smoke detectors should be mounted high on walls or on ceilings. all alarms should be interconnected so when one sounds, the entire house will alarm and alert the residents.
- Ionization smoke alarms are recommended to detect flaming fires. Photoelectric smoke alarms detect smoldering fires. Combination alarms that contain both types of sensors are recommended. Regular monthly testing and battery changes are required at least annually.

Carbon Dioxide Detector

- Carbon dioxide is a colorless odorless gas that binds to the red blood cells and reduces the oxygen level in your blood.
- The installation of carbon dioxide detectors is required in residents that burn natural gas, wood, coal, gasoline, heating oil, and propane. Carbon dioxide is dangerous when it is burned in a confined space like basements, garages, and kitchens. If the alarm sounds, the household should be vacated and the fire department should be called.

Safe Place to Sleep

- Infants should be placed on a firm crib or bassinet surface on their back with a fitted sheet in place. Infants should sleep in the same room as the parents in close proximity but not in the same bed for 1 year ideally or for 6 months at a minimum. The bed should be clear of blankets, bumpers, sheets, and toys.
- Sleeping on sofas, couches, chairs, or recliners is not recommended and is associated with a risk of suffocation.

Avoidance of Secondhand Smoke

- Infants should be kept free from secondhand smoke. Infants exposed to smoke have a higher incidence of upper respiratory infections, ear infections, asthma attacks, and SIDS.
- Any smokers within the household should smoke outdoors.

Safety Restraints in Infant Equipment

- A five-point harness should cover both shoulders along with a strap that extends around the waist and between the legs.

- A five-point harness should be used with all infant equipment including car seats, high chairs, bouncing chairs, and strollers to prevent injury due to dropping and falling. The routine use of a five-point harness results in fewer falls and injuries.

Infant Slings

- The use of slings can provide a safe and comfortable sleeping position for infants. Infant positioning should avoid a curved back position with the chin to the chest and a position in which the face is pushed against the wearer's clothing or body.
- Premature and low-birth-weight babies are at the greatest risk for suffocation.
- Follow the TICKS rule for baby sling safety to reduce the risk of suffocation.

  - **T**ight: The sling should be worn tightly, with the baby in an upright position.
  - **I**n view: The baby's face should be in view at all times.
  - **C**lose enough to kiss: The head should be close enough to kiss at all times.
  - **K**eep the chin off the infant's chest at all times.
  - **S**upport the back, with the infant's back and chest in a natural position at all times.

Clean Environment

- The living environment should be kept clean and hygienic.
- Insist anyone holding the baby first wash their hands. Individuals with flus, colds, or other illnesses should not visit the home and under no circumstances hold the baby. Individuals with cold sores should be cautioned not to make oral contact with the baby.
- Individuals in routine contact with infants should ensure they are up to date with vaccinations including an annual influenza shot.

PROPER THERMAL ENVIRONMENT

Ideally, homes should be kept at a consistent temperature and free from drafts. The ideal temperature is 68°F to 72°F in both the summer and winter months. When temperatures are lower, infants may become chilled and uncomfortable and wake up unnecessarily. Direct air conditioning exposure and supplemental room heaters are not recommended; however, the use of fans to circulate air has been associated with a reduction in SIDS rates.

In preterm babies, the ideal room temperature is 72°F. A warmer room prevents the extra caloric burning that may be induced to maintain a constant temperature in preterm infants. Dressing babies in layers allows baby to maintain adequate heat in colder temperatures. Parents should be reminded to remove extra layers when they come inside.

Fast Facts

When infants are too warm, it increases the risk of SIDS. Parents should be cautioned that wrapping a baby in excessive blankets or clothing can result in overheating.

FAMILY AND ENVIRONMENTAL RISK ASSESSMENT

A comprehensive family and environmental risk assessment should be conducted so healthcare professionals can identify potential stressor and risk factors that can adversely impact the family. Table 27.1 lists risk factors and common interventions that can help reduce stressors for the family (Davidson, Ladewig, & London, 2020).

Table 27.1

Family and Environmental Stressors and Risk Factors		
Risk Factor	**Examples of Associated Risks**	**Interventions**
Inadequate financial resources	Insufficient finances make it difficult to maintain household expenses, purchase infant supplies, and provide for nutritional needs of the family.	Refer for aid for utility assistance, low-cost and subsidized housing alternatives, social service programs, the Women, Infants, and Children (WIC) program, nonprofits for assistance with infant needs, food pantry services, soup kitchens, and homeless shelters for families.
Lack of transportation	Lack of transportation can lead to difficulties maintaining employment, purchasing food and infant care items, obtaining medical care, prescriptions, and accessing social service programs.	Refer for low-cost transportation services, cab or transportation vouchers, bus tokens for public transportation services, andavailable ride-share services for individuals with disabilities.

(continued)

Table 27.1

Family and Environmental Stressors and Risk Factors (*continued*)

Risk Factor	Examples of Associated Risks	Interventions
Access to healthcare	Inability to obtain or maintain healthcare services including preventative care services, immunizations, prenatal care, and well-child visits	Referral to Medicaid, low-cost insurance programs, free or low-cost clinics, and medical services with sliding fee scales. Provide resources including public health clinics, county mental health services, nonprofit organizations providing medical services, and immigrant health clinics.
Neighborhood safety	Residence in an unsafe neighborhood, high-crime areas, or overcrowded living conditions	Review safety strategies, advise against being outdoors at night, encourage neighborhood watch programs, and refer for subsidized housing options in safer neighborhoods.
Unsafe water and sanitation	Residence lacking clean water and adequate sewage services	Notify county of potentially unsafe water sources. Encourage well testing on a regular basis and alerting landlords to faulty water and sewage systems.
Firearms in the home	Presence of weapons or firearms in the household	Advise family of dangers involving gun violence and accidental firearm deaths among children. Encourage all firearms to be stored unloaded in a locked gun safe in a location not accessible to children.

References

Davidson, M. R., Ladewig, P. L., & London, M. L. (2020). *Old's maternal newborn nursing and women's health across the lifespan* (11th ed.). Boston, MA: Pearson Education.

28

Issues in the Home Environment

Family violence can play a significant role in long-term adverse outcomes in infants and children. Family assessments should be performed to identify families at risk for violence and substance abuse.

Community-based postpartum services provide families with invaluable resources to promote health and family wellness. The nurse provides these resources during the postpartum period and at well visits during the first year of life. The health and well-being of infants and children are closely associated with maternal mental health and well-being. Postpartum depression and mood disorder screening are imperative, as 15% to 20% of women develop postpartum depression after the birth of an infant.

During this part of the orientation, the nurse will be able to:

1. Define neglect and child abuse.
2. Review practices to ensure safety when selecting a child care setting.
3. Define sudden unexpected infant death (SUID)
4. List the most common causes of infant injuries in the first year of life.
5. Describe interventions to reduce the risk of sudden infant death syndrome (SIDS).

6. Identify the symptoms associated with postpartum depression.
7. Delineate supportive care measures that can be used for the woman who leaves the hospital without her infant.

CHILD ABUSE

Be aware of the cumulative effects of ongoing family violence. Infants can sense tensions within the home and become fussier and show signs of agitation and crying in the presence of verbal altercations.

Adverse Outcomes of Child Abuse and Neglect

- Mental illness
- Developmental delays
- Alterations in brain development
- Behavioral problems
- Learning disabilities
- Adverse physical health outcomes
- Adolescent and adult substance abuse
- Criminal activity
- Adaptation of abusive behaviors against others
- Victimization
- Poor parenting practices

Numerous behaviors fall under the category of family violence including:

- Intimidation
- Verbal abuse
- Emotional/psychological abuse
- Social abuse
- Economic abuse
- Sexual abuse
- Controlling behaviors

Cumulative exposure to violence is as dangerous as direct acts of more physically threatening violence and harm. Children exposed to violence during infancy up until the age of 3 are more likely to show signs of aggression in early childhood that persists into adolescence and adulthood. Children exposed to family violence are more likely to suffer from adverse psychological symptoms (Harvard University Center of the Developing Child, 2020).

NEGLECT

Child neglect is the failure of a parent or caregiver to provide the care, supervision, affection, and support needed to ensure a child's health, well-being, and safety. Neglect accounts for 78% of all child abuse and is associated with significant physiological and psychological adverse outcomes. Neglect may include physical, emotional, medical, or educational neglect. Infants and children with poor parent–infant attachment are at a risk for ongoing alterations in development including the following (Eichenwald, Hansen, Martin, & Stark, 2017):

- Alterations in physical growth
- Cognitive delays
- Disruption in executive functioning
- Altered self-regulation skills
- Disruptions in stress responses

Physical Abuse

Physical abuse includes any nonintentional injury inflicted upon a child by a parent or caregiver. Physical abuse accounts for 17% of all cases of child abuse (Davidson, Ladewig, & London, 2020).

Fast Facts

If child abuse is ever suspected, immediately report to the county social services agency. Nurses and other healthcare professionals are considered mandatory reporters and must by law report suspected abuse.

Abusive Head Trauma

Abusive head trauma (AHT), also known as *shaken baby syndrome*, occurs as a result of direct blows to the head, dropping or throwing a child, or shaking a child. Head trauma is the leading cause of death in child-abuse cases in the United States. Although any infant can sustain AHT, it occurs more frequently in low-socioeconomic-status families with male infants. Perpetrators are often male caregivers who react as a result of the infant crying.

Symptoms of AHT may include (Centers for Disease Control and Prevention [CDC], 2020):

- Lethargy
- Irritability or lack of smiling or vocalizing

- Vomiting or decreased appetite
- Poor sucking or swallowing
- Rigidity
- Seizures or altered consciousness
- Difficulty breathing
- Unequal pupil size, hemorrhages in the retinas of the eyes, or inability to focus the eyes or track movement
- Skull fractures or swelling of the brain
- Subdural hematomas
- Rib and long-bone fractures
- Bruises around the head, neck, or chest
- Inability to lift the head

Adverse Outcomes Related to AHT

AHT can result in immediate death for the infant. Adverse outcomes related to AHT in infants who survive include:

- Partial or total blindness
- Hearing loss
- Seizures
- Developmental delays
- Intellectual disability or severe intellectual impairment
- Speech and learning difficulties
- Problems with memory and attention
- Cerebral palsy

Fast Facts

If an infant is ever experiencing any symptoms of AHT, immediate medical attention is imperative.

NEWBORN AND INFANT SUPERVISION

The care of newborns and infants is a critical decision for parents. Educate parents to screen potential childcare providers extensively. Childcare options include placement with a family member, placement in an individual's private home, or day care provided in child care centers. Initial steps should focus on finding dependable safe childcare options utilizing the following process:

- Obtain recommendations from healthcare providers and other parents.

- Obtain a background check on the individual and/or facility.
- Check state licensing boards for licensure compliance and complaints and accreditation.
- Meet the individual or visit the child care center in person.
- Ensure the provider is certified in Infant and Child CPR and First Aid.
- Drop in for an unannounced visit.
- Check all references.
- Assess safety procedures, including proper sleep positioning for infants.
- Assess the environment for cleanliness, safety precautions in place, and specific policies and procedures.
- Ask about the longevity of staff members as well as the hiring and screening practices for employees in child care centers.

SUDDEN UNEXPECTED INFANT DEATH

SUID is the death of an infant younger than 1 year of age that occurs suddenly and unexpectedly. After investigation, these deaths may be diagnosed as suffocation, asphyxia, entrapment, infection, ingestions, metabolic diseases, cardiac arrhythmias, trauma (accidental or nonaccidental), or SIDS.

UNINTENTIONAL INJURIES LEADING TO INFANT DEATH

Unintentional injuries are the fifth-leading cause of death in infants younger than 1 year of age. The most common causes of unintentional infant death include the following:

- Infant suffocation
- Motor vehicle-, traffic-related
- Drowning
- Fire/burns
- Poisoning
- Falls
- Other transportation-related causes

Prevention of Infant Injuries

- Avoid having the infant sleep in bed with others.
- Remove extra blankets, pillows, heavy comforters, or toys from the crib.
- Always secure the infant in a rear-facing car seat.

- Ensure home has functioning smoke detectors.
- Test smoke detectors each month.
- Never hold an infant while cooking.
- Never leave a child unattended in a pool or an area containing standing water.
- Never leave an infant on a bed or other elevated surface unattended.
- Use infant gates, window guards, and stair gates to prevent falls.
- Never leave medications in reach of children.
- Dispose of all old medications that are no longer in use.
- Keep all medication in containers with safety tops.
- Make sure food items are properly cut to correct size to prevent choking.

SUDDEN INFANT DEATH SYNDROME

SIDS is the sudden death of an infant younger than 1 year of age that cannot be explained after a thorough investigation, autopsy, death-scene investigation, and a review of the clinical history. It is estimated that there are 2,100 SIDS deaths annually in the United States (CDC, 2020). African Americans and American Indian/Alaskan Natives have double the risk of SIDS (CDC, 2020).

Prevention Strategies for SIDS

- Place the baby on his or her back to sleep.
- Use a firm sleep surface covered by a fitted sheet.
- Baby should sleep in a crib.
- Co-sleeping should be discouraged.
- Soft objects, toys, and loose bedding should not be placed in the crib.
- Secondhand smoke should be avoided completely.
- Breastfeeding during the first year reduces SIDS risk.
- Provide a pacifier that is not attached to a string.
- Avoid overheating the room temperature and overheating the infant by overdressing.

SCREENING AND PREVENTION OF POSTPARTUM DEPRESSION

Postpartum depression affects 15% to 20% of new mothers.

Other postpartum mood and anxiety disorders include postpartum anxiety, postpartum obsessive-compulsive disorder, and postpartum psychosis. Symptoms of postpartum depression vary, but diagnosis is based on the presence of five or more of the following symptoms:

- Depressed mood
- Loss of interest in previously enjoyed activities
- Significant weight loss or appetite change
- Insomnia or hypersomnia
- Loss of energy or fatigue
- Feelings of worthlessness or excessive guilt
- Diminished ability to concentrate
- Suicidal thoughts

Risk Factors for Postpartum Mood Disorders

There are multiple risk factors for postpartum mood disorders; therefore, identify women who are at risk for proper screening. Women with bipolar disorder are at the greatest risk of developing postpartum psychosis and need additional support and assessment during the postpartum period. Risk factors for postpartum mood disorders include:

- Past history of mental health disorder (especially depression)
- Past history of postpartum depression
- Isolation
- Poor social support
- Other stressors (moving, job loss, pregnancy complications, etc.)
- Financial problems
- Marital/relationship issues

Nursing Interventions for Postpartum Mood Disorders

- Perform postpartum depression screening on all women at the postpartum visit.
- Pediatric care providers can also screen women for postpartum mood disorders because they often have prolonged contact with women after the birth.
- Facilities should select a screening tool/instrument for routine use, such as:

  - Edinburgh Postpartum Depression Scale (EPDS)
  - Postpartum Depression Screening Scale (PDSS)
  - Patient Health Questionnaire (PHQ-9)
  - Center for Epidemiologic Studies Depression Scale (CES-D)

- Encourage participation in postpartum and new-mother support groups.
- Refer to postpartum depression support groups.
- Refer to Postpartum Support International.

- Interdisciplinary care management
  - Psychological counseling
  - Medication evaluation
  - Support groups
  - Peer support

POSTPARTUM SUPPORT SERVICES

The postpartum period represents a time of tremendous change for the new family. Adequate postpartum services ensure optimal newborn and family well-being. Families who receive postpartum support services have better outcomes, reduce the risk of maternal postpartum mood disorders, and are more likely to act appropriately if newborn complications occur. Suggested community-based services should include:

- Social support in the postpartum period
- More frequent nursing or social service visits for at-risk mothers
- Availability of use of online support and services
- Interdisciplinary care services
- Assistance from family members at home
- Assistance with child care for older children
- Low-income clinics

Community Resources for PMADS

For some women and families, geographic or lack of family assistance can lead to isolation and the need to obtain all their support from the community. Suggested community-based services should include:

- New mother/infant support classes in the community
- Postpartum depression groups
- Newborn care classes
- CPR Training
- Breastfeeding consultation services
- Breastfeeding support services (La Leche League)
- Support services for new fathers
- Telephone follow-up from care providers
- Nursing or social services home visits
- Low-income clinics

ONLINE SUPPORT

In the age of technology, many new mothers utilize online support systems for an essential network of support. Most nonprofit and maternal–newborn organizations have online resources, which can be accessed at the mother's convenience from her home. These may include contact information, videos, written information, and hotlines where mothers can call to ask questions or access resources. Social media provides a platform for diverse groups of mothers to connect and build a community. Some of these groups are focused in geographic areas and can be utilized to build friendships and access support. Other groups have a specialized focus, such as postpartum support groups, where mothers can connect with others sharing similar issues and needing support. Social groups also have an online presence for mothers to meet other mothers and families. For example, military families can connect with other military families and provide advice and encouragement.

DISCHARGE OF THE MOTHER WITHOUT HER INFANT

The majority of infants are discharged with their parents; however, a small number of women will be discharged without their infants. In most cases, the infant remains hospitalized due to illness or prematurity. A small number of women place their infants for adoption, whereas others have had social services intervention that prohibit the release of the newborn with the mother. Other women may have suffered a fetal demise or neonatal loss, discussed in detail in Chapter 24, Neonatal Ethical Conflicts and Considerations.

Considerations for Women Discharged Without Their Infants

- Consider the psychological implications (sadness, guilt, fear, depression).
- Consider the physical demands of the mother (traveling back and forth to the hospital, pumping breast milk around the clock).
- Support the mother with a hospitalized infant.

  - Encourage frequent visits.
  - Encourage phone calls to check on the infant's status.
  - Support breastfeeding efforts.
  - Facilitate sibling interactions and visitation.
  - Provide an area for parents to rest and sleep.

- Support the mother who relinquishes her infant.

  - Provide mementos, including a photo, crib card, blanket, etc.
  - Encourage participation in support groups.
  - Provide referrals for peer counseling.
  - Provide referrals for counseling support as needed.

References

Center for Disease Control and Prevention. (2020). *Preventing abusive head trauma.* Retrieved from https://www.cdc.gov/violenceprevention/child abuseandneglect/Abusive-Head-Trauma.html

Davidson, M. R., Ladewig, P. L., & London, M. L. (2020). *Old's maternal newborn nursing and women's health across the lifespan* (11th ed.). Boston, MA: Pearson Education.

Eichenwald, E. C., Hansen, A. R., Martin, C. R., & Stark, A. R. (2017). *Cloherty and Stark's manual of neonatal care* (8th ed.). Philadelphia, PA: Wolters Kluwer.

Harvard University Center of the Developing Child. (2020). *Neglect and child abuse.* Retrieved from https://developingchild.harvard.edu/science/deep-dives/neglect/

Index

abdomen, examination of, 58–59
abdominal circumference, 53
abdominal paracentesis, 235
ABR. *See* auditory brainstem
    response method
abstinence screening. *See* neonatal
    abstinence screening
abusive head trauma (AHT), 285
    adverse outcomes, 286
    symptoms, 285–286
ACE. *See* angiotensin-converting
    enzyme inhibitors
acholic stools, 17
acrocyanosis, 54
active acquired immunity, 18, 19
active alert, 272
active sleep, 270
acute kidney injury (AKI), 222
    intrinsic, 222
    postrenal, 222
acyclovir, 162
adefovir, 164
afterload reducers, 115
AHT. *See* abusive head trauma
AKI. *See* acute kidney injury
albinism, 187
albumin, 112
alcohol
    fetal alcohol spectrum disorders,
      169

    -related birth defects, 169
    use, in pregnancy, 168
alcohol-related neurodevelopmental
    disorder, 169
alkaline phosphate, 142
allergies to commercial formulas, 91
ambiguous genitalia, 59–60
American Academy of Pediatrics,
    74
    Refusal-to-Vaccinate form, 264
American College of Medical
    Genetics, 219
Amicar, 240
aminoglycoside, 165
amniocentesis, 248
ampicillin, 124, 165
analgesics, 115, 232
anemia, 156
anesthesia, neonatal, 235–236
angel dust. *See* phenylcyclidine
    (PCP)
Angelman syndrome, 188
angiogram, 212
angiotensin-converting enzyme
    (ACE) inhibitors, 196, 201
antepartum exposures, and
    congenital defects, 185–186
anterior fontanel, 53
antibiotics, 85, 86, 103, 122, 124,
    140, 159, 207, 221, 223, 224

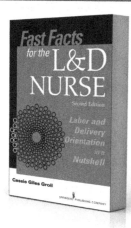
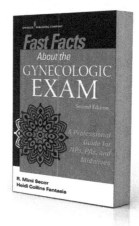
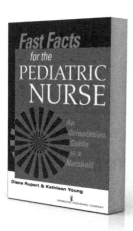
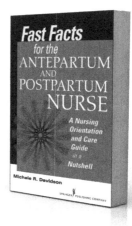